THE ESSENTIAL COOKBOOK FOR MEN

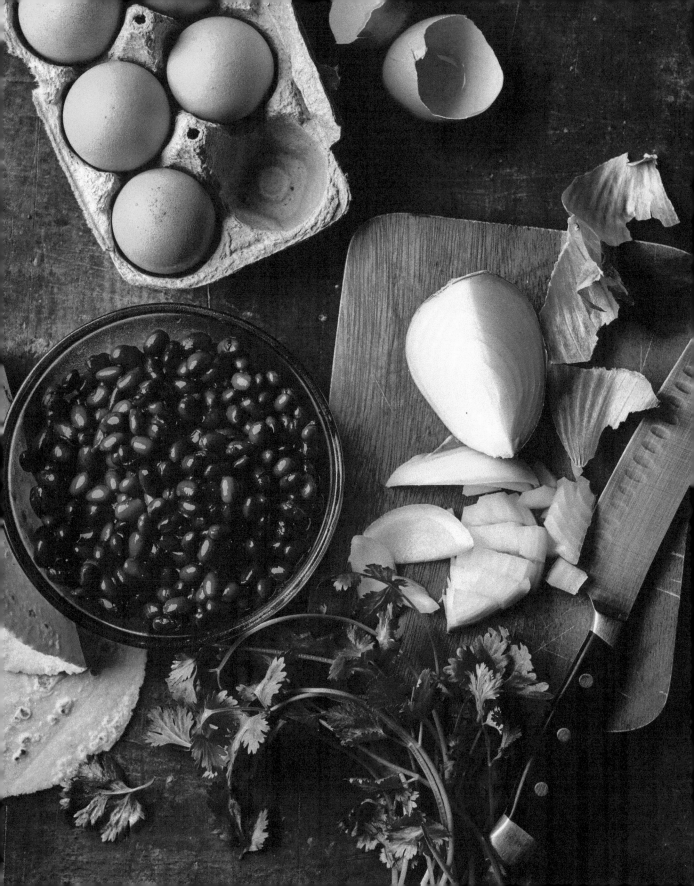

THE ESSENTIAL
COOKBOOK
FOR MEN

85 Healthy Recipes to Get Started in the Kitchen

Manuel Villacorta, MS, RD

Photography by Thomas J. Story

ROCKRIDGE
PRESS

For general information on our other products and services or to obtain technical support, please contact our Customer Care Department within the United States at (866) 744-2665, or outside the United States at (510) 253-0500.

Rockridge Press publishes its books in a variety of electronic and print formats. Some content that appears in print may not be available in electronic books, and vice versa.

Interior and Cover Designer: Brian Lewis

Art Producer: Sue Bischofberger

Editor: David Lytle

Production Editor: Mia Moran

Photography © 2019 Thomas J. Story. Food styling by Karen Shinto.

ISBN: Print 978-1-64152-908-2 | eBook 978-1-64152-909-9

R0

*Thank you, Mamá, for inspiring and teaching me
how to make your delicious recipes.
Learning to cook changed my life.*

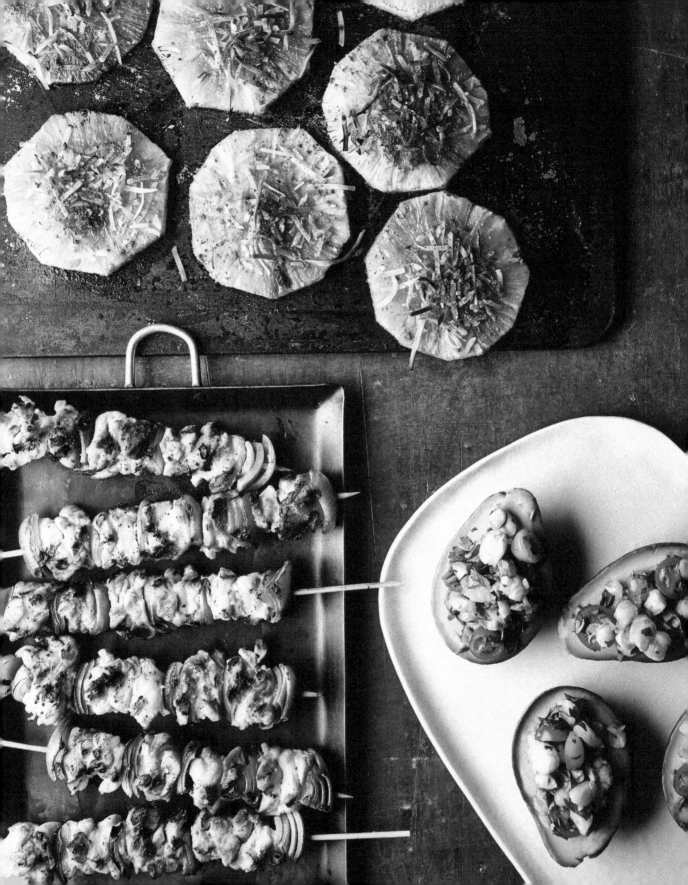

CONTENTS

Chapter Five: **Dinner Mains** 55

Chapter Six: **Basic Sides** 79

Chapter Seven: **Smart Salads (and Dressings)** 89

Chapter Eight: **Desserts** 101

Chapter Nine: **Hearty Snacks** 111

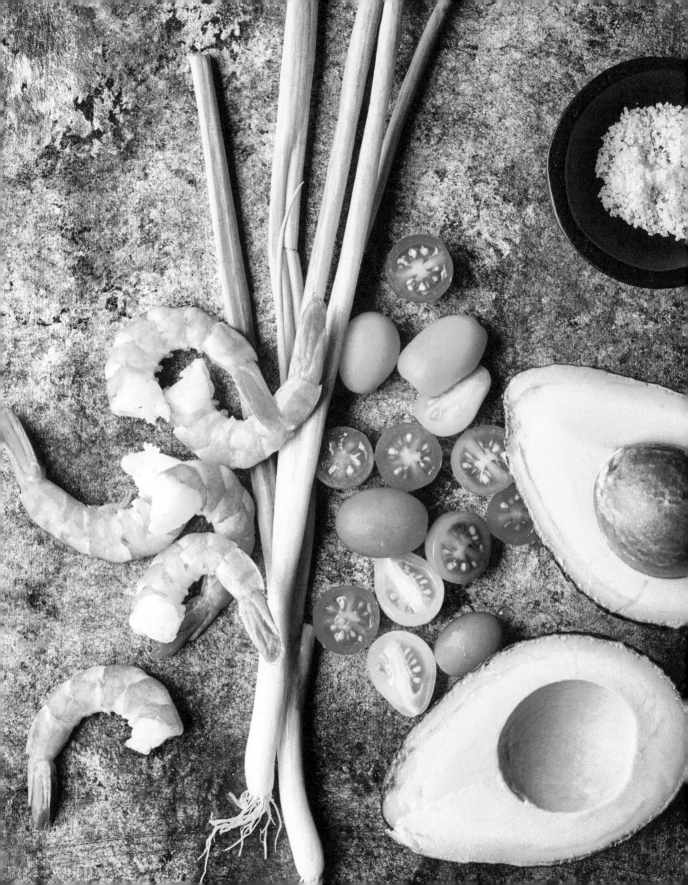

INTRODUCTION

At the age of 20, I moved to the United States from my home in Peru. As a young man whose mother used to cook all of his meals for him at home, I had no idea what I was doing in the kitchen. So, naturally, I went out regularly to eat. Eating out took some adjusting because, back in Peru, we all sat down as a family to have *almuerzo*, which was our regularly scheduled lunchtime. Unlike a typical lunch, it was more like a grand dinner feast. So, going out to have a meal alone and at sporadic times was an odd practice, to say the least.

After a year of living in the US, I missed my mother's cooking and its connection with *almuerzo*, and honestly, I was just tired of eating out. Being from Peru, the food I ate in American restaurants was often unfamiliar. I also realized I was spending way too much money, which is hard for a young foreigner. I wrote a letter to my mother (yes, people wrote letters before there was email and Facebook) and asked her to send me my favorite recipes from home. Not only would home-cooked meals take the stress off of my wallet, I knew I needed to learn to cook if I wanted to enjoy the quality of food—as well as the act of eating and the relationship with food—that I had in my younger years.

Since childhood, I've always wanted to help people. In the wake of my eye-opening American adventure, I enrolled at UC Berkeley to complete an undergraduate degree in premed to follow a healing path. At the same time, I began using my mother's recipes, and I slowly taught myself to cook. It definitely wasn't easy at first, but I quickly figured things out on my own through mistakes and downright culinary failures. For example, I learned that I shouldn't cook meat on the highest setting unless I wanted dry, burned chicken that was like the Sahara in your mouth. My most important lesson was learning how to make food taste better without adding large amounts of fat, sugar, or salt by instead accenting with more herbs and spices.

In any case, food became my primary interest as I was simultaneously learning all about the human body. Quite organically, the two worlds collided. I came to understand that what we eat is at the root of form, function, and disease—the cause and the cure—and that my healing quest would come through food. It was my "aha" moment! It's when I knew my medical path would turn toward dietetics. So, literally, you could say that cooking changed my life. To this end, ever since I became a registered dietitian, I have been promoting cooking at home.

Now I am honored and excited to introduce *The Essential Cookbook for Men* and help guide you through your kitchen, avoiding the mistakes of 20-year-old me. I look forward to sharing my wisdom and culinary skills with you. This cookbook is a delicious way to learn to cook if you are just starting out and will give you skills to last a lifetime. Expect to reboot your gut, improve your total health, and have more energy. Get ready to experience a lifelong journey that will keep you strong, healthy, rejuvenated, and empowered to take control of your health right in your own kitchen.

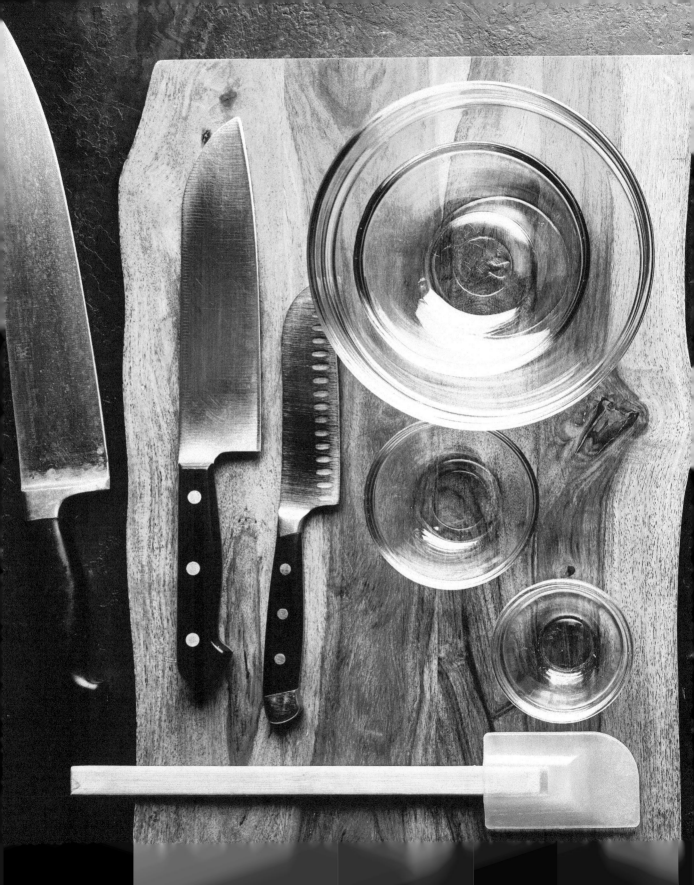

CHAPTER ONE

WELCOME TO YOUR KITCHEN

If you are brand new to cooking, navigating the kitchen might seem overwhelming. The good news? I'm here to help. I always tell clients in my private practice that health starts in the kitchen. That's because *you* are the only one in charge of your ingredients and portions.

GEAR GUIDE

Sometimes when I'm invited to someone's home to cook a meal, I find that I'm out of my element because they don't have the equipment I use to make cooking easy and fun. For example, they may not have the right kind of knife or they may have the wrong type of cutting board. Before you start cooking, I highly recommend that you get the basic tools you'll need to be successful. Here is a guide to the bare essentials, and you can always grow from there as you become more comfortable in your kitchen.

POTS AND PANS (AND LIDS)

SKILLETS- A skillet (also called a frying pan) is essential in the kitchen. This tool is incredibly versatile and is used for a wide range of cooking techniques from frying eggs to making frittatas to sautéing vegetables. I recommend getting a 10- to 12-inch skillet.

POTS- When it comes to pots, I recommend starting with a 4-quart pot with a lid, but you can get a bigger one if you prefer. The 4-quart pot is a good size because it is useful for cooking rice, quinoa, beans, soups, and stews. Many of the recipes in this book should be prepared in this size pot.

ROASTING PANS- A roasting pan is used for cooking at high temperatures, which means less cooking time. This is not only an efficient culinary technique but also a delicious method to cook your food. Roasting pans can be used to roast foods like meat, potatoes, and vegetables and give them a wonderful texture and excellent flavors.

BAKING SHEETS- Baking sheets typically come in a set of three and are very useful in the kitchen. They are perfect to use for meats, vegetables, cookies, and whole meals. One of my favorite recipe types, included in this book, is called sheet pan dinners and makes cooking effortless and cleanup a snap.

SPOONS

Let's keep this very simple. For cooking, as long as you own a ladle (a serving spoon for stews, soups, and other liquid-based foods) and one or two wooden spoons for stirring hot foods, you're in good shape.

CUTTING BOARDS

The two most common types of cutting boards are wooden and plastic. However, wooden cutting boards are my personal favorite. You can choose either one depending on your budget and what feels best for you. Either way, I recommend having at least two cutting boards: one for meat and the other for produce and other foods to prevent cross-contamination (more on that later).

PREP BOWLS

At a minimum, you should have at least three metal or glass bowls, including small, medium, and large sizes. What you use will depend on the quantity of food you are mixing.

KNIVES

There could be an entire chapter just on knives because, believe it or not, they are very complex utensils. While there is a knife for every task in the kitchen, you will mainly be using only three types. The first type is a chef's knife—the most vital knife in your kitchen. It usually has a wide blade that can be 6- to 10-inches long and is used for slicing and dicing fruit, veggies, meats, and much more. The second type is a paring knife, which is smaller and more maneuverable. This makes it ideal for peeling fruits and vegetables. Lastly, you'll need a bread knife, which has a serrated blade intended to be able to cut through soft, delicate bread without crushing it.

How to Use and Care for Knives

Kitchen knives are a nonnegotiable tool in cooking, so it's essential to know how to use them properly. Not only is the correct use of your knives important for safety, but improper use of kitchen knives over time can affect their lifespan. This could be especially important if you invest in an expensive chef's knife or costly set of knives. Keeping your blades "healthy," so to speak, is not only economical but crucial for kitchen safety.

First and foremost, always make sure your knives are sharp. I cannot stress this enough, but the most dangerous tool in the kitchen is a dull knife. When a knife is dull, it doesn't slice through foods smoothly or efficiently. It requires more force to press into the food than you would typically use, and if the knife slips or your hands are in the wrong place, this could lead to a serious injury. Make sure that whatever knives you buy also have a tool for occasional sharpening or get your blades sharpened professionally.

Another important tip is to make sure you are using the correct knife for the job. For example, it isn't practical to use the wide blade of a chef's knife to hull strawberries or peel an apple.

Attempting these tasks could result in higher injury risk (and more labor) than using the easier-to-manage paring knife for the job.

As mentioned on page 3, I recommend the use of wooden and plastic cutting boards in the kitchen. An added benefit of these types of boards is they help preserve your knives. It's been shown that using glass or stone cutting boards have the potential to dull or even damage the blades of knives over time. Use the right type of cutting board, and your knives will thank you. When cleaning knives, never put them at the bottom of a soapy water-filled sink with other dishes. All it takes is for you to forget it is there or someone unaware that it is there to reach in and get cut. You also should never put your knives in the dishwasher. The intense pressure of the water can knock your knives around with other utensils, which can dull them over time. The best way to clean your blades is carefully, by hand, with a sturdy dishcloth or sponge. Finally, accidents do happen. If you do cut yourself with a knife, run the wound under cold water until the bleeding stops, and then apply a bandage. However, if the cut is notably deep and you cannot stop the bleeding even with pressure, you'll want to seek medical attention. Hopefully, however, if you follow my guidelines, this won't be necessary.

STORAGE CONTAINERS

These are a must-have for your leftovers. I recommend buying a set of storage containers found all in one box. This way, you have different sizes for all of your needs. The bigger ones can hold your entrées, the medium ones can hold side items, and smaller ones can be used for sauces and dressings if needed.

APPLIANCES

The essential appliances I recommend are a 64-ounce or larger blender, a small food processor, and an electric pressure cooker or Instant Pot® to help you cook meals in less than thirty minutes. Some of the electric pressure cookers like Instant Pot® offer a feature for slow cooking that will also allow you to slow cook meals, which can be useful for those with limited time.

Other tools you might find useful are an electric hand mixer, immersion blender, spatula, zester or box grater, tongs, measuring cups and spoons, oven mitts, a can opener, and a meat thermometer.

PANTRY ESSENTIALS

When first getting into the habit of doing your own cooking, the upfront cost and tasks of shopping can be a little overwhelming. How do you know you have everything you need? Well, that's why I have a list of what I call "pantry essentials," which are necessary items you should always keep on hand for convenience. Pantry essentials are usually frozen, canned, or dried, which is excellent because they can be stored for a long time without going bad. There are a lot of misconceptions regarding frozen, canned, and dried foods that I will clear up here. I assure you that these products are nutritious and safe to eat. As a registered dietitian and spokesperson for many food commodities, I've had the pleasure of being a guest at many farms, orchards, and fields throughout the United States and have experienced firsthand how foods are grown and processed. I am confident after reading this section you will feel good about keeping your pantry stocked with these gems.

FROZEN

Frozen fruit and vegetables sometimes have an undeserved reputation as being unhealthy. However, I have visited numerous farms and learned that a lot of times frozen produce has more nutritional value than fresh. Let me explain. Imagine you buy a head of broccoli that then sits in your refrigerator for five days before you finally use it in a recipe. During those five days, the vegetable gradually loses some of its nutrition. When vegetables are frozen, however, they are picked at the peak of freshness and frozen very quickly, literally within hours of being taken from the field. Since they are frozen, they retain their nutrients. Another benefit is that frozen produce can be stored for weeks instead of being forgotten in the bottom of your refrigerator and eventually tossed. Frozen fruits and vegetables are often very affordable, which is a plus for anyone's budget. Also, let's not forget proteins. Frozen, cooked meats like chicken strips and meatballs can be lifesavers when you need a meal in a pinch.

CANNED

If frozen produce has a bad reputation, then canned fruit and vegetables have it even worse. Canned fruit, vegetables, and beans are often vilified as containing too much sodium and sugar, having less nutritional value than fresh, and overall being overly "processed." In fact, in many cases, it is the opposite. One good example is tomatoes. Tomatoes contain an antioxidant called lycopene, which has been known to prevent prostate cancer, preserve eyesight, and lower the risk of heart disease. The canning process makes lycopene more bioavailable. This means the body can absorb more lycopene from canned than from fresh tomatoes. And what about them being processed? Again, as I've observed on farms, produce reaches local canneries to be cleaned and diced or sliced before canning within hours after harvest. Food is lightly and quickly heated to create an airtight seal, so the in-season flavor can be enjoyed year-round. Some canned food that I recommend keeping on hand are tomatoes, beans, and fruit. When buying canned food, be sure to buy those with labels indicating low salt or no salt added and fruit in their own juices rather than heavy syrups.

DRIED

Dried fruit has become a bit of a forgotten treasure. One big reason my clients tell me they don't eat enough fruit is that they don't have the time to cut, peel, or prepare it. Other people may not be comfortable with some preparations, such as getting the seeds out of a pomegranate. Fruit often ends up spoiling and is thrown away before my clients can enjoy it, so they are hesitant to purchase more. This is where dried fruit comes into play. One benefit is that dried fruit has a longer shelf life and won't spoil as quickly as fresh fruit. You also don't have to worry about refrigeration, which means dried fruit can be your go-to portable snack. The nutrients are very concentrated in dried fruit because most of the water is removed, so you can get a hefty nutritional boost in a smaller volume than fresh fruit. But not all dried fruit is created equal. I recommend looking for dried fruit that contains no added sugar.

DRIED HERBS AND SPICES

Dried herbs and spices can be an excellent way to add flavor, depth, and even culture to dishes without adding extra calories. In the typical American diet, heavy creams, saturated fats, and refined sugars are often used to please the palate in dishes. However, by using dried spices and herbs, you can elevate your food while keeping it light and healthy. The primary essential herbs and spices to keep in your pantry are sea salt, freshly ground black pepper, garlic powder, onion flakes, oregano, Italian seasoning, and chili powder. Now, if you want to take it to the next level, you can also stock up on ground cinnamon, ground cumin, and turmeric.

OILS, VINEGAR, CONDIMENTS, AND SAUCES

Adding healthy oils and responsibly composed condiments (such as mayonnaise made with avocado oil) are also a great way to flavor your dishes. The healthy recipes in this book will ask for certain oils and sauces to be added, so they must be as nutritionally sound as the main ingredients. Canola oil, for example, is my go-to cooking oil because of its mild flavor, unsaturated fat content, and high smoke point, meaning it will not burn at high temperatures. Another oil I use is extra-virgin olive oil, which is rich in heart-healthy monounsaturated fats. As for sauces, I recommend stocking up on soy sauce, barbecue sauce, mustard, ketchup, and mayonnaise. The best vinegars to keep on hand include balsamic and cider as well as white and red wine.

I am very excited that you will be using these pantry essentials in your cooking and I will show you how to use them to create the delicious dishes in this book.

GROCERY STORE GUIDE: HOW TO SHOP

Knowing how to shop is the key to taking control of your health. When you go out to eat, you may find that it is difficult to discern food quality, fat, sugar, and freshness in what you're consuming. In addition to that, American restaurants typically serve absurdly large portion sizes, way bigger than necessary for a satisfying meal. Unfortunately, since this style of dining out is standard now, we almost always end up overeating, and this is partially due to wanting to get our money's worth. That's where home cooking comes to the rescue. When you handle these variables by buying your own food and preparing it, not only will you experience a smaller hit to your bank account, but you can also radically change your health for the better. That's why I encourage people to get back into the kitchen when looking to take control of their weight and health. If you're reading this book, you've already taken a big first step. However, you won't get far with your cooking if you don't know how to grocery shop—and wisely.

First of all, never go to the store hungry. We've all heard this one before, but it's still true. When you're ravenous and faced with every food product under the sun, your judgment can go south before you know it. Therefore, be aware that the worst time to go grocery shopping is actually right after work. If you go there hungry because you've had a stressful, busy day, you'll forget the healthy products you originally had in mind to buy and grab items that look good. So, always have a snack first, and be sure to bring—and stick to—your grocery list. Grocery lists can be a game changer because not only do they enable you to get in and out faster, but they keep you from impulsively buying things that may not be the best for you.

Another thing I like to tell people is to shop in a familiar store where you're comfortable. This may sound silly, but some people assume that improving their health means changing over to a new, special store, like an organic market. If you choose to shop at such a place, it's fine; however, it's important to know your store layout. Otherwise, you can be overwhelmed and seduced by unfamiliar items, and you may end up buying things that distract you from your health goals. Finally, if you do choose to shop at one of these specialty stores, be sure it is within your budget, so you don't end up discouraged from healthy eating because it seems unaffordable.

Most major grocery stores are set up in the same way. The outer areas usually contain whole foods such as fresh fruits and vegetables, dairy products, and fresh meat. The center aisles hold most of the packaged and processed foods. Unfortunately, you'll find that most people enter their grocery stores and walk right into the latter section first! When you enter the grocery store, I want you to stick to the outer perimeter and know the aisles that contain healthy options, like rice, legumes, whole grains, and pasta. That being said, you definitely shouldn't avoid the center aisles completely because they can also contain foods that are excellent for you such as canned fruit and vegetables. If you're wondering what aisles you should steer clear of altogether, do not even cut through aisles with candies, cookies, and chips if those things are not on your list. Why put yourself through the temptation? Stay focused, and shop smart.

When shopping on a budget, I love to encourage people to visit their local farmers market every once in a while. Seasonal and local produce is usually more affordable, and you also get to support your local farmers! If you buy meats, try buying the whole chicken and break it down yourself. Why? Chicken sold in pieces can be pricier due to the labor cost. What about fruit and vegetables then? As mentioned, canned and frozen foods are part of a healthy diet, as discussed in the pantry essentials section (see page 5). However, you should know, as with meats, you'll find that precut and washed fresh produce is almost always more expensive than a whole plant you can break down yourself.

Also, I would like to remind you about another forgotten treasure—canned fish. Canned fish like tuna, salmon, and mackerel haven't gone anywhere; people have just stopped using it regularly. Canned fish is an excellent cost-efficient way to consume seafood, an ingredient known for being more expensive than other proteins. However, canned fish is more affordable, and it can be stored longer than fresh seafood, which can spoil and be discarded when not used up quickly.

One final tip about shopping on a budget is about buying name brands. Some food products are the same regardless of whether you buy a name brand or generic. One good example of this is dried herbs and spices. I can say with a fair bit of confidence that the garlic powder that is three dollars more because it is a name brand is not significantly better than a generic brand. Keep this in mind when you go for your initial trip to the grocery store to stock your pantry.

How to Make a Grocery List

Having a well-planned grocery list is your best companion when going shopping. Make shopping easier with a list that you can run down and check off as you collect what you need. Not only will you spend less time wandering around, but it can help you stick to your healthy eating plan. So, now that you know the why, let's talk about how to make a winning grocery list.

The first thing you want to do is plan your meals. Pick two or three breakfast and lunch recipes along with perhaps three dinner recipes that you're interested in preparing for the week. Make sure the serving sizes and portions are enough to cover all of the meals you anticipate eating for the week, including leftovers. If necessary, scale the recipe size to suit your needs and adjust the ingredient quantities, so you purchase the right amount of food. Next, go over the ingredients in these recipes and divide them by the categories in the list here. This may seem a bit excessive, but when you organize by categories, all you need to do is go to the corresponding sections in your supermarket. After all, I'm sure you've found yourself in the bread aisle when milk is next on your list, and the dairy section is on the other side of the store. By splitting your ingredients up into these categories, you'll make your supermarket trip much more efficient.

- Produce
- Dairy
- Meats
- Grains
- Canned Goods
- Paper Goods

Another important tip to consider when making your grocery list is to add up the number of ingredients needed in total. For example, there may be multiple recipes in the meal plan that use red onions. By noting the exact amount, you may be able to save money by buying a bag of red onions rather than buying them individually. Additionally, some recipes may require the same type of herb, spice, or seasoning. Since most seasonings will last you for a while, make a note of what you have so that you don't buy more than necessary.

Pay attention to the recipe instructions when you are making your grocery list! Some may call for paper or plastic products such as parchment paper, aluminum foil, or resealable bags. Obviously, these are just as important as the food for executing a recipe successfully, so be sure you include them also. Finally, check your pantry and refrigerator after making your list and cross off any items you already have on hand.

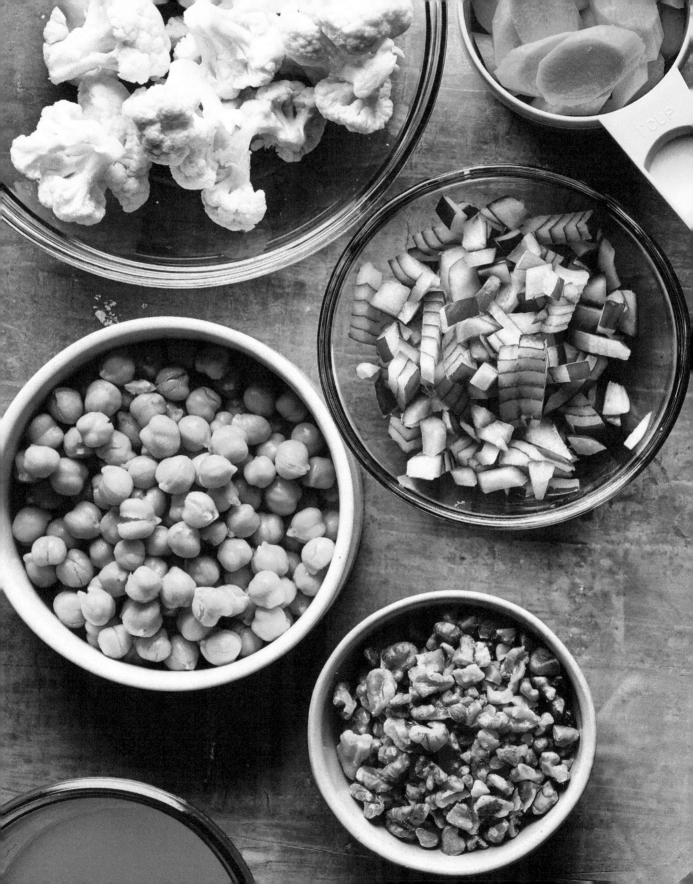

CHAPTER TWO

GET COOKING

Once you have worked up the confidence to start cooking, there are still lessons to learn to keep you both safe and successful. Having healthy recipes in hand is half the battle, but how will you handle your food safely? How should you structure your plate? And what is the best method to keep leftovers or excess ingredients for later? In this section, you'll find all of my tips and tricks for kitchen success, such as:

- How to accurately read and execute your recipes

- The right tools to measure ingredients with precision

- Rules for keeping your kitchen a disaster-free and injury-free zone

- Portion control

- Treating your leftovers with care

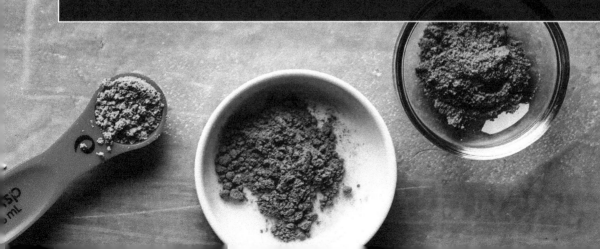

ABOUT THE RECIPES

The recipes in this book have been carefully selected to make your cooking life easier while also optimizing your health. Healthy eating does not have to be time-consuming or expensive. These meals are focused on using unprocessed, whole foods such as fruits, vegetables, and whole grains that will keep you full and satisfied. They also contain fiber for your digestive health, good fats for your heart, and antioxidants to fight inflammation, which is crucial for people of all ages to prevent chronic diseases such as type 2 diabetes, heart disease, and even some cancers.

First things first: How do you read a recipe? This may seem like an obvious question, but when you're first getting started in the kitchen, the simplest things can trip you up. When using a recipe, always read all the way through before touching the first ingredient. It's a good practice to know what steps you are going to take to get to the finished product, so you are prepared for what is next. For example, if a step instructs you to cook something for no longer than two minutes, and it is already on the heat before you set a timer, you could end up with an issue. So make sure you read before you proceed.

In recipes, under the "Ingredients" column, you'll find the measurements for everything you need to make your meal. Typically, ingredients are listed in the order in which they will be used in the recipe. Also, take care to make a note when ingredients need to be prepared first. For example, the recipe may say "red onion, chopped" meaning that this recipe requires a red onion already chopped before you even start cooking.

The "Directions" section will outline what you do with these ingredients and what tools you'll need. This section also outlines whether you need to pre-heat your oven or a skillet while you prepare other components of the recipe. This is another reason to read through the recipe first, so you know what to get ready before you begin. Finally, each recipe will start with how many people it serves, portion sizes when applicable, and prep and cook times.

Timing your shopping well is another good way to ensure success with your recipes. You can either shop the day before and purchase just what you need for one dish, or you can choose one day to do all of your shopping for the week's recipes. Just make sure you don't buy your fresh produce and herbs too far in advance or they may end up spoiling.

FIRE, BLADES, AND GERMS

As important as it is to enjoy your time in the kitchen, it's also crucial to keep yourself safe. Cooking should be approached with a measure of caution and respect because the kitchen does present hazards, but if you stay mindful and diligent, you can minimize any risks.

Since cooking usually requires some form of heat, sometimes intense heat, it's best to be aware of how to stay safe from burns and fires. One thing to remember is never leave food unsupervised, especially if cooking with oil or at very high heat. If you need to step away, turn the burner off before doing so. Furthermore, make sure to clean your stovetop often to prevent grease buildup from catching fire. If a grease fire does happen on your stove, contrary to popular belief, do not throw water or flour on it. Baking soda and/or salt are the most effective ways to extinguish it quickly. If the fire is in a skillet or pan, smother it with a lid and remove it from heat. Finally, if you get a fire in your oven or microwave, keeping the door closed will eventually smother the fire. Another great idea is to keep a fire extinguisher in your kitchen or near the kitchen.

To prevent burns, always use an oven mitt or pot holder when taking things out of the oven or when using metal pots and pans. Do not use paper towels or dish towels because they are not sturdy enough to hold very hot vessels. Also, be sure to always keep the handles of pans turned inward to prevent accidental bumps, which could result in nasty (and hot!) spills. Finally, be sure to stand back with your face away from the pot when you remove a lid or open the oven door to prevent steam burns.

Next up is pathogens, namely the germs that cause food poisoning. If you are cooking for yourself, your family, or houseguests, you want to serve them some yummy food, not a foodborne illness. The most common causes of food-borne illness are cross-contamination, unsafe food handling, and undercooked food. Fortunately, there are simple steps you can take to prevent all of these.

First, always use a different cutting board to cut your raw meat than the one you use for produce or wash your cutting board in hot, soapy water between uses. Pathogens are prevalent in raw meat, so when handling it, be sure to wash your hands before you touch anything else, including kitchen equipment. Try using a meat thermometer to check that foods are thoroughly cooked and pathogens have been killed off. Finally, do not thaw food on your kitchen counter. Thaw in the refrigerator, under cold running water, or in the microwave.

HOW TO MEASURE

You probably didn't know that liquid and dry ingredients use different tools for precise measurement—and that's okay! We're going to go over the correct way to measure different ingredients to make sure that your recipes turn out deliciously accurate.

Measuring cups are usually sold in a set of increments that includes ¼, ⅓, ½, and 1 cup. These are what you want to use for measuring dry ingredients such as flour, sugar, or cocoa. Dry measurement cups are designed to be leveled off from the top for accuracy.

As for wet ingredients, like water, milk, and broth, they should preferably be measured in a glass measuring cup, one with a spout and a handle. This is preferred because wet ingredients are typically called for in larger quantities than dry ingredients, and also the glass cup allows you to look through and see how much you have in there.

Lastly, you have measuring spoons which are usually sold in a set of increments that includes ⅛ teaspoon, ¼ teaspoon, ½ teaspoon, 1 teaspoon, ½ tablespoon, and 1 tablespoon. These are great for ingredients that are only needed in small quantities and can be used to measure both wet and dry ingredients.

PORTION CONTROL

As time has gone on, our plates have become bigger and bigger, resulting in larger portion sizes. Furthermore, our plate composition is skewed, so there is a less favorable balance between fruit, vegetables, protein, and carbs.

Keeping all of these components in balance is critical for maintaining a healthy metabolism, higher energy levels, and hunger control. Therefore, try to follow these steps to build your plate to ensure you're eating foods in optimal proportions for health:

1. Have the right size plate. Studies have shown that the larger the plate, the more food you will pile on. Plates that are 8 to 9 inches in diameter will help you feel like your plate is full without overeating.

2. Use your measuring cups. Using these utensils allows you to know exactly how much you are eating at each meal. This is also a handy method to keep track of your portions for accurate record-keeping.

3. Learn how to serve. Knowing how to design your plate is crucial. First, half of the plate should be a colorful mix of nonstarchy vegetables, such as broccoli, cauliflower, carrots, tomatoes, asparagus, and/or green leafy vegetables. One-quarter of the plate should be a superfood carbohydrate such as quinoa, sweet potatoes, beans, lentils, brown rice, and/or black rice. Then the most important part, which is protein! This macronutrient should be included in all of your meals. The last quarter of the plate should be a lean protein such as chicken, salmon, lean pork, or tofu.

LEFTOVERS

When cooking you're bound to have leftovers eventually, which is convenient and cost-effective. However, you want to handle your leftovers with care so you don't expose yourself to foodborne illness or end up trashing all of your hard-earned work in the kitchen.

First, before refrigerating your leftovers, be sure to seal them in storage containers with a lid or cover them with airtight packaging such as plastic wrap to keep bacteria out and prevent food from becoming dry and unappetizing. Leftovers can be kept in the refrigerator for three to four days. Make sure your refrigerator temperature is 40°F or below to prevent the growth of pathogens. If you need to keep leftovers longer, freeze them for three to four months. Keep in mind, though, that the longer leftovers are frozen, the more they may lose flavor. When arranging your containers with leftovers in your refrigerator, make sure air can still circulate properly. Without proper circulation, your refrigerator may have issues keeping a safe temperature.

Lastly, my mother always told me that leftovers are just meal prep for the prepared. If you have trouble meal prepping or planning, simply double your dinner recipe. Then, last night's healthy dinner can become tomorrow's healthy lunch. So easy!

Read Those Food Labels

Food labels can be a powerful tool if you know how to read them, so let's go over what you'll find on food packaging labels.

Any food label has a section called **Nutrition Facts**. It's important to know that the data listed here is for one serving, so also look for how many servings there are per container. Nutrition facts lists information amount total fat, saturated fat, trans fat, cholesterol, sodium, total carbohydrates, fiber, sugar, and protein. Amounts for each are displayed as weight in grams and as the percentage of the USDA's daily recommend allowance. Below this list, you'll find a bar offering daily recommend allowances for specific vitamins as well. After those sections, we get to the list of **ingredients**. Always keep in mind that this list is organized by the amount of each ingredient by weight, so if a sugar is listed first, just know you're about to consume an awful lot of unhealthy sugar.

But not all sugar is unhealthy. Recently, some labels have started listing natural sugars and added sugars. For example, the amount of sugar in a serving of yogurt may be just as high as the amount of sugar in a small dessert, but that does not mean they are equal. The sugars in dairy and whole fruit are natural sugars that come with healthy nutrients and fibers, whereas the sugars found in candies and sodas are added sugars that can cause a whole range of health issues if consumed in excess. If you see an ingredient in the list that ends with "-ose" or is some form of syrup, this product likely has added sugars and the food should be consumed sparingly. Also keep in mind that if the list of ingredients is very long or contains things you cannot pronounce, you're probably looking at a highly processed food that is just not as healthy as a whole food. A good rule to follow is to stick to packaged foods that contain no more than five ingredients.

Finally, always take note of the **expiration date** stamped somewhere on the package. Stores cannot sell items past these dates, and it's recommended that you don't eat anything past its expiration dates. Wasting food can be a bummer so, to avoid this, time your grocery trips wisely and store older products in front of fresher products in your pantry and fridge to make sure you use them first.

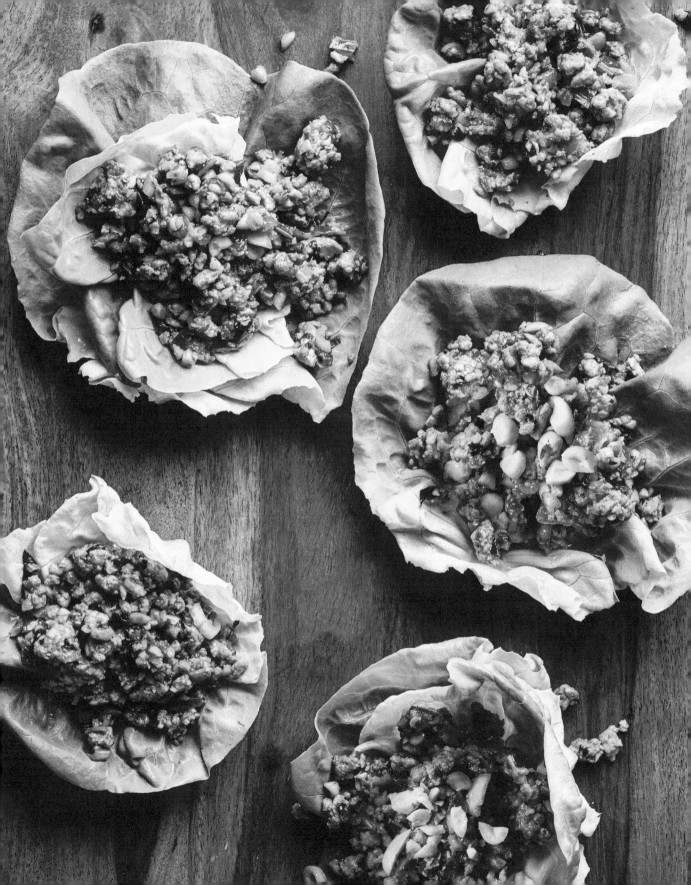

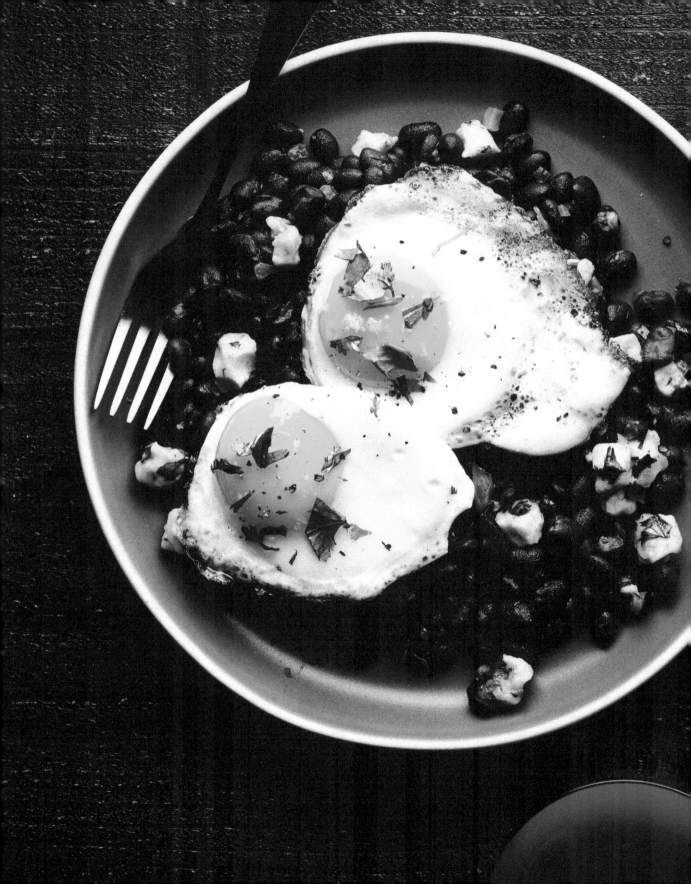

CHAPTER THREE

BREAKFASTS

There's nothing that can boost a new-to-the-kitchen chef's confidence more than starting his day off right by making breakfast for himself. These breakfast recipes allow for lots of variety and range from savory to sweet, so you can play around with whatever you are in the mood for. Having a balanced breakfast that includes complex carbohydrates, high-quality protein, and good fats helps give you energy and mental clarity and boosts your metabolism for the day. If you're new to the kitchen, I recommend starting with the recipes with the least ingredients and saving the more complex ones for when you have more time.

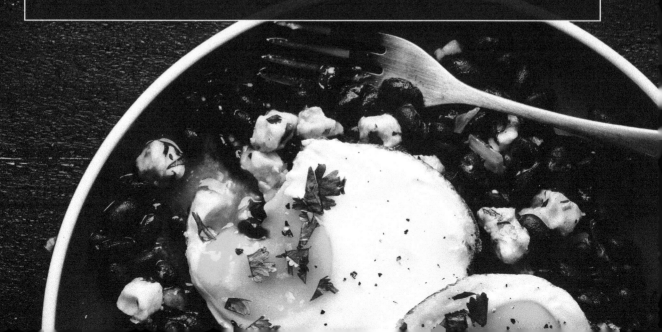

OVERNIGHT OATS TO GO

PREP TIME: 5 MINUTES, PLUS 6 HOURS TO SOAK | SERVES 4 (SERVING SIZE: 1 CUP)
30 MINUTES OR LESS | ONE POT | VEGETARIAN

This delicious breakfast on the go is quick to throw together and is an easy way to start your day. Oats are a good source of soluble fiber, which slows down digestion and keeps you full. Any dried or fresh fruit or nuts can be added to this recipe with great results.

4 cups dried oats

6 cups whole milk (or milk of choice)

1 cup prunes, chopped

½ cup walnuts, chopped

2 teaspoons ground cinnamon

¼ teaspoon sea salt

1. Stir together the oats, milk, prunes, walnuts, cinnamon, and salt in a sealable container and allow the oats to soak at least 6 hours or longer overnight in the refrigerator.

2. Stir well before eating.

CHEF'S NOTE: Once the oats are soaked, separate the mixture into containers so you can have it ready in the morning and take it to go throughout the week.

NUTRITION TIP: Research suggests that eating 5 to 6 prunes each day may help prevent bone loss. Prunes have both potassium and magnesium and are a source of vitamin K. All three of these nutrients are important for bone health.

Per serving: Calories: 728; Total fat: 28g; Sodium: 327mg; Carbohydrates: 102g; Fiber: 13g; Sugar: 35g; Protein: 25g

CARROT CAKE SMOOTHIE

PREP TIME: 7 MINUTES | SERVES 1
30 MINUTES OR LESS | ONE POT | VEGETARIAN

I get inspired when my clients take action and become creative in the kitchen after I've coached them. This recipe comes from my client Roman Rodriguez, who shared it with me. I love it so much that I'm sharing it with you now.

1 cup whole milk (or milk of choice)

1 cup sliced carrots (1 to 2 carrots)

1 tablespoon chia seeds

2 teaspoons ground cinnamon

1 teaspoon finely chopped peeled fresh ginger

1 scoop protein powder* (whey, soy, pea, or rice)

Note: To provide 25 grams of protein

1. Pour the milk in a blender, then add the carrots, chia seeds, cinnamon, ginger, and protein powder. Blend until smooth.

2. Chill in the refrigerator until cold and serve.

CHEF'S NOTE: You can make this smoothie the night before and have it ready for breakfast.

NUTRITION TIP: Chia seeds have plant-based omega-3 fatty acids. Omega-3s can help fight inflammation and heart disease. Add them to any smoothie for an extra boost.

Per serving: Calories: 384; Total fat: 11g; Sodium: 356mg; Carbohydrates: 34g; Fiber: 11g; Sugar: 17g; Protein: 37g

WARM CHOCOLATE BANANA
PEANUT BUTTER SMOOTHIE

PREP TIME: 5 MINUTES | SERVES 1
5 INGREDIENTS | 30 MINUTES OR LESS | ONE POT | VEGETARIAN

On a cold morning, this smoothie will put you in the right mind-set to start your day. Nourishing and delicious, the combination of chocolate, banana, and peanut butter is unbeatable. It is almost like having dessert for breakfast, and you might be inspired to create other warm smoothies when the temperature drops outside.

1 cup whole milk (or milk of choice), warmed in the microwave for 1 minute

1 (7-inch) banana

1 tablespoon peanut butter

1 tablespoon cocoa powder

1 scoop chocolate protein powder* (whey, soy, pea, or rice)

*Note: To provide 25 grams of protein

1. Pour the milk in a blender, then add the banana, peanut butter, cocoa powder, and protein powder.

2. Blend until smooth and serve.

CHEF'S NOTE: Bananas come in all sizes. If you can only find extra-large bananas, consider using half and saving the rest for an afternoon snack.

NUTRITION TIP: Use natural peanut butter without added sugars.

Per serving: Calories: 483; Total fat: 17g; Sodium: 333mg; Carbohydrates: 46g; Fiber: 6g; Sugar: 26g; Protein: 39g

POWER PACKED PARFAIT

PREP TIME: 5 MINUTES | SERVES 1
5 INGREDIENTS | 30 MINUTES OR LESS | ONE POT | VEGETARIAN

Studies show that nuts and seeds can help people control their weight. When added to this parfait, they'll help increase your satiety and hold you over until lunch. If blueberries aren't your jam, feel free to substitute another berry, such as sweet strawberries and raspberries or tart blackberries.

1 cup 2% plain Greek yogurt
¾ cup fresh blueberries
1 tablespoon chopped walnuts

1 teaspoon chia seeds
1 tablespoon honey

Layer the ingredients in a bowl as follows: half of the yogurt, half of the blueberries, half of the walnuts, and half of the chia seeds. Do another layer in the same order and finish the parfait with a drizzle of honey.

CHEF'S NOTE: To take this recipe on the go, make it in a mason jar with a lid instead of a bowl. Throw the jar in your backpack or lunch box for an easy breakfast or snack you can enjoy at work. Eat this snack within three hours of packing it or refrigerate until you are ready to eat it.

NUTRITION TIP: Greek yogurt has more protein than regular yogurt.

Per serving: Calories: 359; Total fat: 11g;
Sodium: 113mg; Carbohydrates: 44g; Fiber: 5g;
Sugar: 37g; Protein: 25g

PUMPKIN SPICED OATMEAL

PREP TIME: 5 MINUTES | COOK TIME: 10 MINUTES | SERVES 4 (SERVING SIZE: 1 CUP)
30 MINUTES OR LESS | ONE POT | VEGETARIAN

When you're craving a holiday treat, this is the recipe for you. Pumpkin pie spice contains all the flavors found in a classic pumpkin pie, like nutmeg, cinnamon, and ginger. The warm fragrance wafting from the simmering oats will make you think of crisp fall days and evenings spent relaxing in front of a crackling fire.

2½ cups whole milk (or milk of choice)
1½ cups rolled oats
¼ teaspoon sea salt

¼ teaspoon pumpkin pie spice
½ cup pumpkin purée
¼ cup roasted pumpkin seeds

1. In a medium saucepan, stir together the milk, oats, salt, and pumpkin pie spice. Cook over medium heat until the oats are softened, about 5 minutes.

2. Stir in the pumpkin purée and cook, stirring occasionally, for another 5 minutes until the mixture has thickened. Mix in the pumpkin seeds and serve.

CHEF'S NOTE: Use old-fashioned dried oats instead of instant or quick oats because they have more texture.

NUTRITION TIP: Pumpkin purée is packed with beta-carotene, which is good for skin and eye health. If you have leftover pumpkin, you can add it to quick breads, muffins, or smoothies.

Per serving: Calories: 235; Total fat: 8g; Sodium: 222mg; Carbohydrates: 32g; Fiber: 4g; Sugar: 9g; Protein: 10g

MEDITERRANEAN-STYLE SCRAMBLED EGGS

PREP TIME: 5 MINUTES | COOK TIME: 10 MINUTES | SERVES 1
30 MINUTES OR LESS | VEGETARIAN

This tasty breakfast uses whole eggs so you get the goodness of both the yolk and the white. The yolk contains most of the nutrition in an egg, including protein, vitamin D, and an essential nutrient called choline, which is good for brain health. Many Americans don't get enough choline, so tuck into this savory, satisfying meal often.

1 teaspoon extra-virgin olive oil
3 large eggs
1 tablespoon chopped fresh basil

1 tablespoon chopped sun-dried
    tomatoes (not packed in oil)
8 kalamata olives, sliced
1 tablespoon feta

1. Heat the olive oil in a 10-inch skillet over medium heat.

2. Whisk together the eggs, basil, sun-dried tomatoes, and olives in a medium bowl until well mixed.

3. When the oil is hot , reduce the heat to medium low, pour in the egg mixture, and let it sit for about 10 seconds. Then use a heatproof rubber spatula to sweep lines from one edge of the pan to the other, drawing the eggs into large fluffy segments. Repeat from a new point in the skillet after a few seconds, turning the curds over from the top to the bottom in a scooping motion. Continue this technique until the eggs are mostly set but slightly undercooked, about 1½ minutes. (They keep cooking from skillet to plate.)

4. Add the feta. Mix well. Let sit for 30 seconds while gently stirring to combine.

5. Serve.

CHEF'S NOTE: Serve with whole-grain pita or toast if desired.

NUTRITION TIP: You don't need to add salt because feta, olives, and sun-dried tomatoes are already salted.

Per serving: Calories: 400; Total fat: 33g; Sodium: 862mg; Carbohydrates: 8g; Fiber: <1g; Sugar: 1g; Protein: 21g

LATINX-STYLE FRIED EGGS

PREP TIME: 5 MINUTES | COOK TIME: 7 MINUTES | SERVES 1
30 MINUTES OR LESS | ONE POT | VEGETARIAN

This is a hearty breakfast high in fiber due to the beans. Fiber keeps you full and helps maintain gut health. This recipe is also packed with protein, so it is the perfect way to start an active day. For a more substantial meal, you could tuck the whole recipe into whole-wheat pita bread or wrap in a tortilla.

2 teaspoons canola oil, divided
2 tablespoons finely chopped onion
1 (15-ounce) can black beans, rinsed and drained
1 tablespoon chopped fresh cilantro

2 ounces queso fresco, cubed
2 large eggs
Sea salt
Freshly ground black pepper

1. Heat 1 teaspoon of oil in a medium skillet over medium heat. Add the onion and sauté until translucent, about 1 minute. Add the beans and cilantro and sauté for 30 seconds. Stir in the queso fresco and sauté for another 30 seconds. Transfer the mixture to a plate and set aside.

2. Heat the remaining 1 teaspoon of oil in the same skillet over medium heat. Crack the eggs into the skillet and fry until the whites are completely set and the yolks start to thicken, about 3 minutes.

3. Remove the skillet from the heat and slide the eggs over the bean mixture. Season to taste with salt and pepper.

4. Serve.

> **CHEF'S NOTE:** You can substitute feta or your favorite cheese for the queso fresco.

Per serving: Calories: 798; Total fat: 35g; Sodium: 464mg; Carbohydrates: 73g; Fiber: 19g; Sugar: 5g; Protein: 49g

BROCCOLI EGG PARMESAN MUFFINS

PREP TIME: 5 MINUTES | COOK TIME: 25 MINUTES | SERVES 4 (SERVING SIZE: 3 MUFFINS)
5 INGREDIENTS | VEGETARIAN

As a Fruit and Vegetable Ambassador in Action for the Produce for Better Health Foundation, I help them promote the Have a Plant campaign. My job is to encourage the consumption of fruits and vegetables of all kinds: fresh, dried, or frozen. The goal is for you to eat a plant every day! Therefore, you will see lots of plants included in the recipes in this book to help you reach that goal.

Nonstick olive oil cooking spray
2 cups chopped frozen broccoli, thawed in microwave for about 2 minutes and drained
12 large eggs

3 ounces shredded Parmesan
¼ teaspoon freshly ground black pepper
Sea salt

1. Preheat oven to 350°F. Coat a 12-cup muffin tin with olive oil spray.

2. Evenly divide the broccoli between the muffin cups.

3. Crack the eggs into a large bowl and stir in the Parmesan, pepper, and salt.

4. Evenly divide the egg mixture between the muffin cups leaving a ½-inch space at the top.

5. Bake for 20 to 25 minutes, until the muffins are puffed and lightly browned.

6. Serve.

CHEF'S NOTE: Use foil or paper muffin liners for easy cleanup. The muffins keep well in the refrigerator for up to 4 days.

NUTRITION TIP: Most frozen vegetables are flash-frozen at peak ripeness, so they are highly nutritious.

Per serving: Calories: 325; Total fat: 20g; Sodium: 587mg; Carbohydrates: 5g; Fiber: 1g; Sugar: 2g; Protein: 28g

SWEET POTATO CRÊPES

PREP TIME: 10 MINUTES | COOK TIME: 25 MINUTES | SERVES 4 (SERVING SIZE: 2 CRÊPES)
5 INGREDIENTS | VEGETARIAN

These crêpes are a special creation of my friend Alejandro Pinot. I love them so much that I was compelled to include the recipe in this book. I hope you enjoy them as much as I do. For a real treat, I love eating them with a drizzle of honey on top.

1 (15-ounce) can sweet potato purée
2 cups whole milk (or milk of choice)
4 large eggs

2 cups all-purpose flour
Nonstick cooking spray

1. Whisk together the sweet potato, milk, and eggs in a large bowl until very well blended.

2. Spoon the flour into the wet ingredients 2 tablespoons at a time, whisking well after each addition until all the flour is used.

3. Heat a medium skillet over low heat. Lightly coat with cooking spray. Using a ½-cup measure, scoop the batter into the skillet, tilting the skillet to spread the batter out very thinly. Cook each side for about 1½ minutes.

4. Transfer the finished crêpe to a plate and cover with a clean kitchen towel to keep warm.

5. Repeat with the remaining batter.

6. Serve.

> **CHEF'S NOTE:** If you want to impress your significant other, whip up a batch of these tempting crêpes or try the batter in a waffle maker following the manufacturer's instructions.

Per serving: Calories: 461; Total fat: 9g; Sodium: 215mg; Carbohydrates: 77g; Fiber: 4g; Sugar: 19g; Protein: 19g

WALNUT FIG YOGURT BREAD

PREP TIME: 15 MINUTES | COOK TIME: 45 MINUTES
SERVES 10 (SERVING SIZE: 1-INCH-THICK, 3-OUNCE PORTIONS)
VEGETARIAN

Whether you go to school or work, I recommend starting your day with a solid and balanced breakfast. A meal like that not only gives you a substantial amount of carbohydrates and protein, it also contains a measure of good fats. This hearty, fried fruit and nut studded bread provides the right combination of good carbs and fats to support a healthy lifestyle.

Nonstick cooking spray

1½ cups all-purpose flour

1½ cups dry instant oats (1 minute quick)

¼ cup brown sugar

1 teaspoon ground cinnamon

1 teaspoon baking powder

1 teaspoon baking soda

1 teaspoon sea salt

1 cup 2% plain Greek yogurt

½ cup whole milk (or milk of choice)

2 large eggs

2 tablespoons canola oil

2 teaspoons vanilla extract

½ cup chopped dried figs

½ cup chopped walnuts

1. Preheat oven to 350°F.

2. Coat a 9-inch loaf pan with cooking spray and set aside.

3. In a medium bowl, stir together the flour, oats, brown sugar, cinnamon, baking powder, baking soda, and salt until well mixed. Set aside.

4. In a large bowl, whisk together the yogurt, milk, eggs, oil, and vanilla extract until well blended.

5. Gently whisk the flour mixture into the egg mixture until just combined. Stir in the figs and walnuts.

6. Spoon the batter into the prepared loaf pan and place in oven on the middle rack. Bake for 45 minutes until golden brown. Place a toothpick in the center and if it comes out clean, it is done.

7. Cool the loaf in the loaf pan, pop it out after 5 minutes, and cool on a rack.

8. Serve when cooled.

CHEF'S NOTE: You can enjoy this bread warm. Refrigerate the leftover bread. Next time you eat a slice, warm it in the oven or toaster.

NUTRITION TIP: To make a well-balanced breakfast, pair this bread with a cup of kefir. Kefir is a liquid fermented food like yogurt that provides a good source of protein.

Per serving: Calories: 250; Total fat: 10g; Sodium: 392mg; Carbohydrates: 35g; Fiber: 3g; Sugar: 10g; Protein: 8g

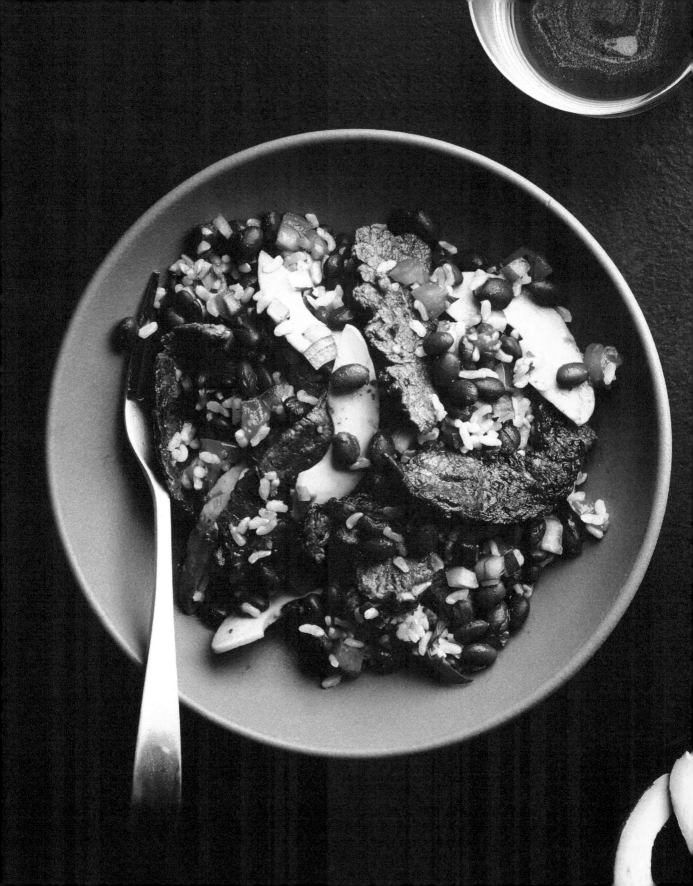

CHAPTER FOUR

LUNCH: SANDWICHES, SOUPS, AND BOWLS

As men, we shouldn't be afraid to carry a lunch box. When I first moved to the United States and was living with American roommates, I would grab a handful of cereal for breakfast while running out the door, and I would scarf down cold sandwiches or get takeout for lunch. Not only did I gain weight, but I lacked energy (along with money) due to eating too much takeout. Many of the lunch recipes here are quick and make multiple servings so you can have leftovers to pack a winning lunch and take control of your health.

AVOCADO EGG TOMATO SANDWICH

PREP TIME: 5 MINUTES | SERVES 1
5 INGREDIENTS | 30 MINUTES OR LESS | ONE POT | VEGETARIAN

There are many different ways to hard-boil an egg, but I thought I would impart the method I have used for years: Put eggs in a single layer in a small pot and cover them by about 1½ inches with cold water. Bring the pot to a boil and then start a timer set for seven minutes. When the timer goes off, take the pot off the heat, drain eggs, and place them immediately in a bowl of ice water.

½ avocado, pitted, peeled, and sliced

2 slices whole-grain bread

1 hard-boiled egg, sliced

½ medium tomato, sliced

1. Put the sliced avocado on one piece of bread and the egg slices on top.

2. Add the sliced tomato and the second piece of bread and enjoy.

CHEF'S NOTE: If you take this sandwich for a to-go lunch, bring the tomato slices in a separate container and add just before eating so the sandwich isn't soggy.

NUTRITION TIP: Squeeze lime juice on the other half of the avocado before storing it to prevent the fruit from turning brown.

Per serving: Calories: 455; Total fat: 22g; Sodium: 414mg; Carbohydrates: 55g; Fiber: 17g; Sugar: 10g; Protein: 21g

CHICKEN AVOCADO WRAP

PREP TIME: 5 MINUTES | SERVES 1 (MAKES 2 ROLLS)
5 INGREDIENTS | 30 MINUTES OR LESS | ONE POT

This is an easy recipe to take on the go and is very quick to prepare. A wrap is an excellent alternative to a sandwich and perfect for lunch at work or school. Lavash is a soft, unleavened flatbread similar to a tortilla but made from wheat. It is popular in the Middle East and western Asian countries.

½ avocado, pitted, peeled, sliced, and divided
2 (10-by-8-inch) pieces whole-grain lavash
Sea salt

2 tablespoons chopped fresh cilantro, divided
4 ounces sliced cooked chicken, divided

1. Arrange half of the avocado slices on a third of the short end of the lavash. Sprinkle the fruit with a pinch of salt and half of the cilantro.

2. Arrange half of the chicken on top of the avocado.

3. Starting from the avocado side, roll the lavash into a roll and cut the wrap in half diagonally.

4. Repeat with the remaining ingredients to make a total of 2 rolls.

5. Serve.

CHEF'S NOTE: Wrap the rolls securely in aluminum foil if taking this tasty wrap to go.

NUTRITION TIP: Adding fresh herbs like cilantro enhances the flavor of foods without the need to add too much salt.

Per serving: Calories: 456; Total fat: 24g; Sodium: 1,228mg; Carbohydrates: 36g; Fiber: 18g; Sugar: <1g; Protein: 45g

PINEAPPLE ROASTED PORK SANDWICH

PREP TIME: 5 MINUTES | COOK TIME: 12 MINUTES | SERVES 6
5 INGREDIENTS | 30 MINUTES OR LESS | ONE POT

If you're a fan of Hawaiian flavors, this is the sandwich for you. Sweet pineapple pairs naturally with savory roasted pork, so whip up this recipe when entertaining a group of friends or for a casual family event. You can substitute canned pineapple slices packed in juice, but you will have to cut the slices into two thinner ones to get the right width.

Nonstick cooking spray

2 pounds boneless pork top loin chop, thinly sliced

1 teaspoon sea salt

½ teaspoon freshly ground black pepper

1 whole pineapple, peeled and cut into ¼-inch-thick slices

6 (6-inch) French rolls

1. Preheat oven to 400°F. Coat a large roasting pan with cooking spray.

2. Place the pork in the pan and sprinkle with the salt and pepper.

3. Remove the hard center core of each pineapple round using a paring knife and arrange the pineapple slices in a single layer on top of the pork.

4. Bake for 12 minutes or until the internal temperature of the pork is 145°F.

5. Let the pork rest until cool enough to handle.

6. Place one piece of pork and 1 to 2 pieces of pineapple inside each French roll.

7. Serve.

CHEF'S NOTE: If you don't want to make a sandwich, serve the roasted pork and pineapple without the bread. To create a meal, add rice or quinoa and pair it with a salad.

NUTRITION TIP: Pork is a protein that is budget friendly, healthy, simple to prepare, and easy to find in any grocery store. Just look for your favorite lean cuts in the meat case—many of these cuts meet the USDA's guidelines for "lean meat," which means they have less than 10 grams of fat per serving.

Per serving: Calories: 529; Total fat: 18g; Sodium: 894mg; Carbohydrates: 52g; Fiber: 3g; Sugar: 9g; Protein: 39g

STIR-FRY BEEF SANDWICH

PREP TIME: 10 MINUTES | COOK TIME: 17 MINUTES | SERVES 4 (6 CUPS, FILLED WITH 1½ CUP PER SERVING)
30 MINUTES OR LESS | ONE POT

This recipe is savory and filling for anyone who enjoys the flavor of onions and peppers. It might remind you of the famous Philly cheesesteak sandwich without the melted cheese topping.

1 tablespoon canola oil, divided

1½ pounds beef round strips

1 medium onion, thinly sliced

1 teaspoon minced garlic

½ red bell pepper, sliced

½ teaspoon sea salt

¼ teaspoon freshly ground black pepper

4 (6-inch) French rolls

1. Heat ½ tablespoon of oil in a medium skillet over medium heat. Add the beef, sauté for about 5 minutes, and set aside.

2. Heat the remaining ½ tablespoon of oil, add the onion, and sauté for 7 minutes or until softened.

3. Add the garlic, bell pepper, salt, and black pepper and sauté for another 5 minutes.

4. Add the cooked beef to the vegetable mixture and mix well.

5. Divide the beef mixture into four portions and place inside French rolls and serve.

CHEF'S NOTE: The stir-fry beef mixture yields 6 cups, so each sandwich is filled with 1½ cups per serving. Assemble the sandwiches right before eating so the rolls do not get squishy. Canola oil is one of the best cooking oils for stir-frying due to its high smoke point, meaning it will not burn as you are cooking.

NUTRITION TIP: Bell peppers have a lot going for them nutritionally. They're low in calories and an excellent source of vitamins A and C.

Per serving: Calories: 567; Total fat: 15g; Sodium: 835mg; Carbohydrates: 43g; Fiber: 2g; Sugar: 1g; Protein: 62g

WHITE BEAN CEVICHE LETTUCE CUPS

PREP TIME: 10 MINUTES | SERVES 2
30 MINUTES OR LESS | ONE POT | VEGAN

This is an inspired vegan take on classic lime-infused ceviche. Instead of raw fish and seafood, the base of this recipe is hearty beans. White beans are an excellent protein source as well as a healthy carbohydrate that is rich in fiber. Fiber is crucial for both digestive health and heart health.

1 (15-ounce) can white beans, drained and rinsed
½ medium red onion, thinly sliced
¼ cup diced red bell pepper
2 tablespoons chopped fresh cilantro

1½ tablespoons freshly squeezed lime juice
½ teaspoon sea salt
⅛ teaspoon freshly ground black pepper
1 head butter lettuce

1. Mix together the beans, onion, bell pepper, cilantro, lime juice, salt, and black pepper in a medium bowl until well combined.

2. Carefully remove the outer leaves of the lettuce and place 1 to 2 together to form a sturdy cup.

3. Spoon the bean mixture into the lettuce cups and serve.

CHEF'S NOTE: You can store any leftovers for up to 3 days in the refrigerator.

NUTRITION TIP: Canned beans contain all of the nutrition of soaked and cooked dry beans with none of the prep work. This product is an easy way to add protein and bulk to a meat-free lunch.

Per serving: Calories: 206; Total fat: 1g; Sodium: 596mg; Carbohydrates: 35g; Fiber: 12g; Sugar: 5g; Protein: 12g

ZESTY CHICKPEA PITA PACKETS

PREP TIME: 10 MINUTES | SERVES 1
30 MINUTES OR LESS | ONE POT | VEGETARIAN

Pita bread is an easy and portable way to carry all sorts of delicious, healthy ingredients like this citrusy chickpea creation. It is best to stuff the pitas just before eating if the filling is juicy or has a generous spoon of sauce. You don't want a soggy meal! If you want to add a little crunch to the dish, toast the pita before spooning in the filling.

1 (15-ounce) can chickpeas, drained and rinsed

2 (7-inch) celery stalks, minced

3 tablespoons avocado oil mayonnaise

2 tablespoons chopped fresh parsley

2 tablespoons freshly squeezed lemon juice

½ teaspoon sea salt

⅛ teaspoon freshly ground black pepper

1 whole-wheat pita, split in half

1. Mix together the chickpeas, celery, mayonnaise, parsley, lemon juice, salt, and pepper in a medium bowl until well combined.

2. Fill each pita half with the chickpea mixture and enjoy.

CHEF'S NOTE: Parsley adds a pretty green color to any dish and enhances the Middle Eastern flair of this delicious meal.

Per serving: Calories: 843; Total fat: 30g; Sodium: 1,933mg; Carbohydrates: 119g; Fiber: 28g; Sugar: 17g; Protein: 33g

MOO SHU PORK LETTUCE CUPS

PREP TIME: 10 MINUTES | COOK TIME: 11 MINUTES | SERVES 4 (SERVING SIZE: ½ CUP OF
PORK MIXTURE AND 2 BUTTER LETTUCE LEAVES)
30 MINUTES OR LESS | ONE POT

This is a great recipe for fans of Chinese flavors, and the seasonings of classic moo shu pork—scallions, soy sauce, ginger, and garlic—are found in these tasty lettuce cups. Ginger and garlic make a fragrant combo when sautéed with the pork. And if you want to create a more traditional version, add a scrambled egg to the filling.

1 tablespoon canola oil
½ medium red onion, chopped
1 pound extra-lean ground pork
1 tablespoon minced garlic
1 teaspoon minced peeled fresh ginger
½ cup cilantro, chopped

4 scallions, chopped (whiter and green parts)
2 tablespoons low-sodium soy sauce
2 tablespoons hoisin sauce
½ cup crushed peanuts
1 head butter lettuce

1. Heat the oil in a medium skillet over medium heat. Add the onion and sauté for about 2 minutes.

2. Add the pork, garlic, and ginger and sauté for about 7 minutes or until the pork is no longer pink.

3. Stir in the cilantro, scallions, soy sauce, hoisin sauce, and peanuts and cook for another 2 minutes.

4. Carefully remove the outer leaves of the lettuce and place 1 to 2 together to form a sturdy cup.

5. Spoon the pork mixture into the lettuce cups and serve.

CHEF'S NOTE: You can store any leftovers for up to 5 days in the refrigerator.

NUTRITION TIP: Peanuts are nutritious and a traditional Chinese garnish, so you will find them added to everything from seafood to salads.

Per serving: Calories: 322; Total fat: 18g; Sodium: 478mg; Carbohydrates: 12g; Fiber: 3g; Sugar: 5g; Protein: 31g

CHICKEN MANGO RAINBOW WRAP

PREP TIME: 5 MINUTES | SERVES 2
30 MINUTES OR LESS | ONE POT

This colorful wrap uses both fruit and vegetables to accent the chicken and create a filling lunch. Mango has a fresh, almost piney flavor that is perfect with earthy cabbage. If your mango is not perfectly ripe, try shredding it on the large side of a box grater. This recipe is not only delicious, it is also a feast for the eyes.

4 ounces cooked chicken breast, chopped (see page 63)
½ cup avocado oil mayonnaise
½ cup mango, cubed

½ cup shredded cabbage
¼ cup shredded carrots
2 (10-by-8-inch) pieces whole-wheat lavash bread

1. Stir together the chicken, mayonnaise, mango, cabbage, and carrots in a medium bowl until well mixed.

2. Divide the ingredients evenly between the two pieces of lavash bread. Spread the mixture on one half of the lavash bread. Roll lengthwise starting at the edge where the mixture was placed.

3. Cut in half and enjoy.

CHEF'S NOTE: Buy shredded cabbage and carrots to make this even easier to prepare.

NUTRITION TIP: Even though mangos are sweet, they have a low glycemic index of 50, making it a diabetic-safe food. Studies have also found that regular consumption of mangos can aid in the reduction of waist size and reduce blood glucose in both men and women.

Per serving: Calories: 591; Total fat: 54g; Sodium: 1,123mg; Carbohydrates: 23g; Fiber: 8g; Sugar: 7g; Protein: 22g

TURKEY BASIL PATTY SANDWICH

PREP TIME: 10 MINUTES | COOK TIME: 7 MINUTES | SERVES 4 (MAKES 4 HAMBURGERS)
30 MINUTES OR LESS

Sweet summer basil goes great with sautéed turkey, and the scallions add flavor and punch. Use whole-wheat hamburger buns for a meal with extra fiber and satiety. This herbed turkey mixture can be formed into tempting meatballs and pan-seared with the same method as the burgers. Just increase the cooking time by about 5 minutes per batch and take care to reach an internal temperature of 165°F.

1 pound ground turkey

½ cup finely chopped scallions, green and white parts (about 4)

¼ cup finely chopped fresh basil

½ teaspoon sea salt

¼ teaspoon freshly ground black pepper

Nonstick cooking spray

4 hamburger buns

1. In a medium bowl, mix together the turkey, scallions, basil, salt, and pepper until well combined.

2. Using a ½ cup measuring cup, divide the mixture into 4 portions and shape into patties.

3. Lightly coat a large skillet with cooking spray and set over medium heat. Add the patties and cook them 3 minutes on one side. Flip them over, cover the pan, and cook them for another 4 minutes or until the internal temperature reaches 165°F.

4. Transfer the burgers to the buns and serve.

> **CHEF'S NOTE:** Add your favorite toppings to your burgers such as cucumbers, lettuce, and tomatoes.

Per serving: Calories: 295; Total fat: 11g; Sodium: 598mg; Carbohydrates: 24g; Fiber: 1g; Sugar: 3g; Protein: 26g

EGG AND APPLE SANDWICH

PREP TIME: 10 MINUTES | SERVES 2
30 MINUTES OR LESS | ONE POT | VEGETARIAN

Apple is an unexpected yet refreshing ingredient in this egg salad. The combination of celery, apple, and tangy yogurt is similar to the classic Waldorf salad so it should be no surprise this filling is delicious. The avocado oil is very rich in healthy fats, lutein, and antioxidants, and is milder tasting than mayo made with olive oil.

3 hard-boiled eggs, chopped (page 34)
1 (6-inch) celery stalk, chopped
½ cup diced apple
2 tablespoons 2% plain Greek yogurt
1½ tablespoons finely chopped red onion

1 tablespoon avocado oil mayonnaise
¼ teaspoon sea salt
⅛ teaspoon freshly ground black pepper
4 slices whole-grain bread

1. Mix together the eggs, celery, apple, yogurt, onion, mayonnaise, salt, and pepper in a medium bowl.

2. Evenly divide the egg filling between 2 slices of bread, spreading it out, and top with the remaining bread slices.

3. Serve.

CHEF'S NOTE: Super fresh eggs are hard to peel. To test the freshness of your eggs, place a whole egg in a bowl of water and if it floats, it is an older egg.

NUTRITION TIP: Pair this sandwich with fruit or salad of choice for a more balanced meal.

Per serving: Calories: 419; Total fat: 17g; Sodium: 799mg; Carbohydrates: 51g; Fiber: 11g; Sugar: 13g; Protein: 23g

CHICKEN MEATBALL BROWN RICE SOUP

PREP TIME: 20 MINUTES | COOK TIME: 15 MINUTES
SERVES 4 (SERVING SIZE: 2 CUPS OF SOUP AND 3 MEATBALLS)

Stock-based soups are both filling and low calorie. Slowly simmering the meatballs in the stock creates an incredibly rich broth, and the brown rice adds bulk and texture to the meal. Brown rice is a whole grain and a healthy carbohydrate source. You could use barley or farro instead for a tasty variation.

For the meatballs

2 pounds ground chicken
1 green bell pepper, diced
½ cup diced red onion

1 teaspoon sea salt
½ teaspoon freshly ground black pepper

For the soup

8 cups low-sodium chicken stock
6 (7-inch) celery stalks, sliced
2 (7-inch) carrots, sliced

1 teaspoon sea salt
½ teaspoon freshly ground black pepper
2 cups cooked brown rice

To make the meatballs

Mix together the chicken, bell pepper, onion, salt, and black pepper in a large bowl. Use a ⅓ cup measuring cup to form meatballs about 2 inches in diameter. Set aside.

To make the soup

1. Pour the stock into a 4-quart stockpot and bring to a boil over high heat. Add the celery, carrots, and the meatballs and simmer for 15 minutes or until the meatballs are cooked through and the vegetables are tender.

2. Stir in the brown rice and season the soup with salt and pepper.

3. Serve.

> **CHEF'S NOTE:** For an easier time making the meatballs, wet your hands before handling the meat to avoid it sticking.
>
> **NUTRITION TIP:** Serve this soup with a side salad for an extra dose of phytonutrient-rich veggies.

Per serving: Calories: 543; Total fat: 26g; Sodium: 2,144mg; Carbohydrates: 34g; Fiber: 5g; Sugar: 5g; Protein: 12g

ROASTED TOMATO SOUP

PREP TIME: 10 MINUTES | COOK TIME: 55 MINUTES | SERVES 4 (SERVING SIZE: 1½ CUPS)

Roasting tomatoes brings out their flavor without adding extra calories or fat. The high heat caramelizes the sugars in the fruit, creating a depth of flavor that is exceptional. Using canned tomatoes instead of fresh for this recipe is an added convenience and reduces prep time.

2 (28-ounce) cans no-salt-added whole plum tomatoes, drained

1 tablespoon extra-virgin olive oil

1 medium red onion, chopped

2 red bell peppers, chopped

1 (15-ounce) can artichoke hearts, drained and chopped

1 cup low-sodium chicken stock

2 teaspoons dried basil

2 teaspoons paprika

1 teaspoon sea salt

1 tablespoon chopped fresh basil

1. Preheat oven to 500°F. Spread the tomatoes in a 16-inch roasting pan and roast for 10 minutes. Remove from oven and set aside.

2. Heat the oil in a large saucepan over medium-high heat, add the onion, and sauté for about 5 minutes or until the onion becomes translucent.

3. Stir in the roasted tomatoes, bell peppers, and artichoke hearts. Sauté for 5 more minutes.

4. Add the stock, dried basil, paprika, and salt. Bring the soup to a boil and then reduce the heat to low. Cover and let simmer for 30 minutes.

5. Remove the soup from the heat, stir in the fresh basil, and let cool for 5 minutes. Once cooled, transfer the soup to a blender or use an immersion blender to purée until smooth.

6. Serve.

CHEF'S NOTE: This soup will last in the refrigerator for 5 days. Make a batch at the beginning of the week for several days' worth of lunches.

NUTRITION TIP: Add a side salad with your protein of choice and a piece of whole-grain bread for a well-rounded meal.

Per serving: Calories: 165; Total fat: 5g; Sodium: 886mg; Carbohydrates: 30g; Fiber: 8g; Sugar: 14g; Protein: 6g

SIRLOIN STEAK MUSHROOM SOUP

PREP TIME: 8 MINUTES | COOK TIME: 15 MINUTES | SERVES 4 (SERVING SIZE: 4 CUPS)
30 MINUTES OR LESS | ONE POT

This recipe will activate your fifth taste receptor, umami. The umami receptor senses glutamate, inosinate, and guanylates. This recipe contains all three! Foods rich in glutamate are tomatoes, mushrooms, and cheese. Inosinate is found in meats such as sirloin steak, and guanylate is found in mushrooms.

8 cups low-sodium beef stock
1 pound sirloin steak, cubed
2 (7-inch) carrots, sliced
1 white onion, diced

3 (7-inch) celery stalks, sliced
8 ounces cremini mushrooms, sliced
1 bunch Swiss chard, sliced
Sea salt

1. In a 4-quart stockpot over medium-high heat, stir together the stock, steak, carrots, onion, celery, and mushrooms.

2. Bring the soup to a boil and then reduce the heat to medium and simmer for 10 minutes.

3. Stir in the chard and simmer for another 5 minutes.

4. Season to taste with salt and serve.

CHEF'S NOTE: Just before serving the soup, give it a good stir so that all ingredients are well distributed.

NUTRITION TIP: When mushrooms are grown in sunlight, they become rich in vitamin D, which is essential for bone and heart health.

Per serving: Calories: 316; Total fat: 7g; Sodium: 1,326mg; Carbohydrates: 18g; Fiber: 6g; Sugar: 6g; Protein: 47g

GINGER CILANTRO CHICKEN SOUP

PREP TIME: 8 MINUTES | COOK TIME: 15 MINUTES | SERVES 4 (SERVING SIZE: 4 CUPS)
ONE POT

This is a Thai-inspired take on comforting chicken noodle soup. Ginger has been shown to support the body's natural defense against disease by activating T cells, which are an essential part of your immune system since they destroy infected cells. If you're not comfortable cutting up a whole chicken, ask your butcher to do it.

1 whole chicken

8 cups water

1 (3-inch) piece fresh ginger, peeled and thinly sliced

1 red onion, chopped

2 (7-inch) celery stalks, sliced

2 (7-inch) zucchini, sliced

2 (7-inch) carrots, peeled and sliced

2 teaspoons sea salt

¼ teaspoon freshly ground black pepper

½ cup cilantro, chopped

1. Using a sharp chef's knife, remove the skin from the whole chicken and cut into eighths. Make sure the chicken breasts are cut in half. In total, you should have two drumsticks, two thighs, and four chicken breasts. Wings are optional to keep.

2. In a 4-quart pot over medium heat, combine the chicken, water, ginger, and onion and bring to a simmer. Simmer, uncovered, for about 35 minutes (skim off foam every so often).

3. Add the celery, zucchini, and carrots to the pot and cook for another 15 minutes.

4. Season with the salt and pepper.

5. Add the cilantro and mix well.

6. Serve.

> **NUTRITION TIP:** By replacing the noodles with vegetables, you get added nutrition, and the soup will be very low carb.

Per serving: Calories: 256; Total fat: 6g; Sodium: 1,335mg; Carbohydrates: 8g; Fiber: 3g; Sugar: 4g; Protein: 42g

CHERRY TOMATO AVOCADO GAZPACHO

PREP TIME: 15 MINUTES, PLUS 1 HOUR TO CHILL | SERVES 4 (SERVING SIZE: 1½ CUPS)
30 MINUTES OR LESS | ONE POT | VEGAN

Each element of this bright soup adds flavor and texture. The avocado provides a rich creaminess, the cherry tomatoes and red pepper burst with sweetness, and the onion and chili paste produce a hint of heat and sharpen the overall taste. Serve chilled in the summertime for a refreshing lunch.

1 pound red cherry tomatoes
1 medium cucumber, peeled and chopped
1 ripe avocado, pitted and peeled
1 red bell pepper, chopped
½ medium red onion, chopped
½ cup low-sodium vegetable stock

¼ cup fresh parsley, chopped
¼ cup white wine vinegar
1 tablespoon aji amarillo or other chili paste
1 tablespoon freshly squeezed lime juice
1½ teaspoons sea salt
1 teaspoon garlic, minced

1. Place the tomatoes, cucumber, avocado, bell pepper, onion, stock, parsley, vinegar, chili paste, lime juice, salt, and garlic in a blender and purée until the desired consistency is reached.

2. Refrigerate the soup for 1 hour before serving to allow the flavors to mellow.

CHEF'S NOTE: The longer this veggie-packed soup sits, the more flavorful it gets.

Per serving: Calories: 141; Total fat: 8g;
Sodium: 1,004mg; Carbohydrates: 17g; Fiber: 6g;
Sugar: 7g; Protein: 3g

FARRO WITH VEGETABLE CHICKEN BOWL

PREP TIME: 10 MINUTES | COOK TIME: 15 MINUTES | SERVES 4 (SERVING SIZE: 1½ CUPS)
30 MINUTES OR LESS

Farro is an ancient whole grain derived from wheat. It is a tasty alternative to brown rice and can be mixed with almost anything with stellar results. Try this delicious bowl for a filling lunch.

6 cups water

1 tablespoon plus ½ teaspoon extra-virgin olive oil, divided

8.8 ounces or about 2 cups dry quick-cooking farro

1 yellow onion, sliced

2 (7-inch) carrots, sliced

1 cup prunes, chopped

½ cup walnuts, chopped

1 teaspoon balsamic vinegar

¼ teaspoon freshly ground black pepper

Sea salt

1 pound cooked chicken breast, chopped (see page 63)

1. In a one-quart stockpot, combine the water and ½ teaspoon of oil. Bring to a boil over high heat and stir in the farro. Reduce the heat to medium and simmer for 10 minutes. Drain and set aside.

2. While the farro is cooking, heat the remaining 1 tablespoon of oil in a large skillet over medium heat. Add the onion and carrots and sauté for 2 minutes.

3. Stir in the prunes, walnuts, vinegar, pepper, and salt. Cook for another 2 to 3 minutes.

4. Stir in the cooked farro and chicken and cook for 2 more minutes to allow the flavors to meld.

5. Serve.

CHEF'S NOTE: Refrigerate the leftovers for up to 5 days.

NUTRITION TIP: With the entire wheat kernel intact, farro is a good source of B vitamins and fiber.

Per serving: Calories: 738; Total fat: 19g; Sodium: 88mg; Carbohydrates: 105g; Fiber: 16g; Sugar: 20g; Protein: 44g

QUINOA SPINACH PESTO BOWL

PREP TIME: 10 MINUTES | COOK TIME: 20 MINUTES | SERVES 4 (SERVING SIZE: 1 CUP)
30 MINUTES OR LESS | VEGAN

Did you know that quinoa is not a grain but a seed from the same family as spinach? Quinoa grows in the Andes Mountains of South America, mainly in Peru and Bolivia, and has been a staple in these regions for over 5,000 years. You'll love this dish.

1 tablespoon extra-virgin olive oil

3 cups fresh spinach leaves, lightly packed

2 cups fresh basil leaves, lightly packed

¼ cup diced red onion

¼ cup low-sodium vegetable broth

¼ cup pine nuts, toasted

¼ teaspoon sea salt

¼ teaspoon freshly ground black pepper

4 cups Basic Quinoa (page 80)

1. Heat the oil in a large skillet over medium heat. Add the spinach, basil, and onion and sauté for 2 minutes or until the spinach is wilted.

2. Transfer the spinach mixture to a blender or food processor and add the vegetable broth, pine nuts, salt, and pepper. Blend until desired consistency.

3. Serve the cooled quinoa with the pesto and with the protein of your choice.

CHEF'S NOTE: Pair this recipe with your protein of choice. For example, crack a couple eggs on top for a savory breakfast.

NUTRITION TIP: Substituting pasta with quinoa increases the nutrition value of this meal. Quinoa is known to have all nine essential amino acids, so it is considered a complete protein.

Per serving: Calories: 344; Total fat: 14g; Sodium: 196mg; Carbohydrates: 48g; Fiber: 10g; Sugar: 5g; Protein: 11g

TRI-COLORED POTATO CILANTRO FUSION WITH CHICKEN BOWL

PREP TIME: 10 MINUTES | COOK TIME: 20 MINUTES | SERVES 4 (SERVING SIZE: 2¼ CUPS)
30 MINUTES OR LESS

Peru boasts of over 5,000 kinds of potatoes. When you visit the open markets in Peru, you see a sea of multicolored potatoes. It's quite attractive and fascinating. The Peruvian purple potato, which is available here in the United States, has more antioxidants than most other potatoes.

3 pounds small tri-colored potatoes
4 (7-inch) celery stalks, finely diced
1 cup 2% plain Greek yogurt
½ cup chopped fresh cilantro
¼ cup finely diced red onions

1 tablespoon extra-virgin olive oil
1 tablespoon freshly squeezed lemon juice
1 teaspoon sea salt
¼ teaspoon freshly ground black pepper
5 ounces cooked chicken breast

1. Place potatoes in a large pot and cover with cold water. Bring to a boil over high heat, then reduce to low and simmer for 20 minutes, or until the potatoes are soft. Drain the potatoes and set aside to cool for about 10 minutes, then cut them in half.

2. In a large bowl, stir together the celery, yogurt, cilantro, onions, oil, lemon juice, salt, and pepper. Add the potatoes.

3. Add the chicken on top of the salad and serve.

CHEF'S NOTE: Depending on the size of the potatoes, you can leave them whole or cut them into smaller bite-sized pieces. I like a chunkier bite, so cutting in half works for me.

NUTRITION TIP: Substituting regular white potatoes for colored potatoes adds more antioxidants.

Per serving: Calories: 366; Total fat: 6g; Sodium: 725mg; Carbohydrates: 59g; Fiber: 7g; Sugar: 9g; Protein: 20g

SALMON POKE BROWN RICE BOWL

PREP TIME: 5 MINUTES | COOK TIME: 5 MINUTES | SERVES 4
(SERVING SIZE: 5-OUNCE SALMON WITH 1½ CUPS RICE EDAMAME MIXTURE)
30 MINUTES OR LESS | ONE POT

A lot of people think the only healthy choice is fresh salmon, but canned fish offers the same great benefits, such as a hefty amount of omega-3 fatty acids and protein. An excellent choice for canned salmon is Alaskan wild salmon because of its clean taste and deep color.

4 cups cooked brown rice

2 cups frozen edamame, thawed and heated according to package instructions

2 tablespoons sesame seeds

1 tablespoon low-sodium soy sauce

20 ounces canned wild-caught salmon, drained

½ cup sliced scallions (green parts only)

1. Mix the rice and edamame in a medium bowl until well combined. Add the sesame seeds and soy sauce and stir to combine.

2. Divide the rice mixture evenly into four bowls. Top each with about one-fourth of the salmon. Garnish with the scallions.

3. Serve.

> **CHEF'S NOTE:** Divide the rice mixture into different bowls before adding the salmon or add the salmon when ready to eat. Refrigerate leftovers up to 5 days.
>
> **NUTRITION TIP:** Edamame is full of fiber and vitamin K.

Per serving: Calories: 735; Total fat: 32g; Sodium: 1,298mg; Carbohydrates: 56g; Fiber: 8g; Sugar: 1g; Protein: 59g

LATINX STEAK BOWL

PREP TIME: 15 MINUTES | COOK TIME: 10 MINUTES | SERVES 4 (SERVING SIZE: CUP OF RICE
AND BEAN MIXTURE, ½ CUP PICO DE GALLO, 4 OUNCES OF STEAK, AND ¼ AVOCADO)
30 MINUTES OR LESS

This recipe is easy and quick, especially if you keep a batch of pico de gallo in your refrigerator as a healthy accent for your meals. Use leftover brown rice, open a can of beans, and you have a meal in 15 minutes flat. This is a filling meal with a Latinx touch, and it's quite delicious!

For the pico de gallo

3 tomatoes, diced

¼ cup diced red onion

¼ cup chopped fresh cilantro

1 jalapeño pepper, seeded and diced

1 tablespoon freshly squeezed lime juice

½ teaspoon sea salt

For the bowl

1 teaspoon canola oil

1 pound flank steak, thinly sliced

½ teaspoon sea salt

¼ teaspoon freshly ground black pepper

2 (15-ounce) cans black beans, drained and rinsed

2 cups cooked brown rice

1 avocado, pitted, peeled, and sliced

To make the pico de gallo

In a medium bowl, stir together the tomatoes, onion, cilantro, jalapeño, lime juice, and salt and set aside.

To make the bowl

1. Heat the oil in a large skillet over medium heat. Add the steak, season with the salt and pepper, and sauté for 10 minutes.

2. Remove the skillet from the heat and stir in the beans, rice, avocado, and pico de gallo.

3. Distribute the mixture into bowls and serve.

CHEF'S NOTE: Don't worry if the meat starts to turn crunchy and brown. This is how I make steak, the Latinx way.

NUTRITION TIP: The amount of pico de gallo and avocado in this dish gives you at least a serving of vegetables.

Per serving: Calories: 580; Total fat: 16g; Sodium: 660mg; Carbohydrates: 68g; Fiber: 15g; Sugar: 5g; Protein: 40g

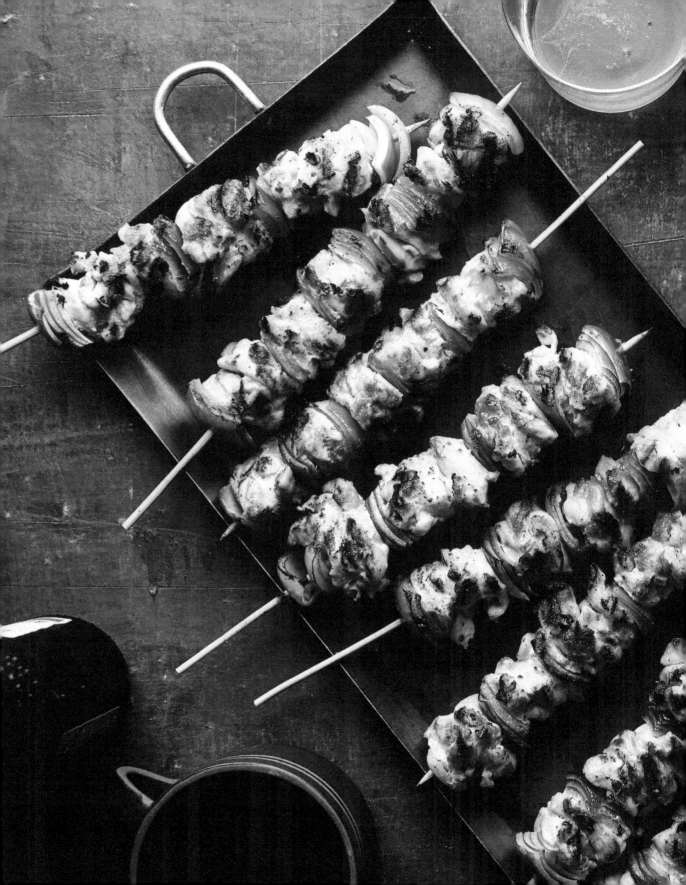

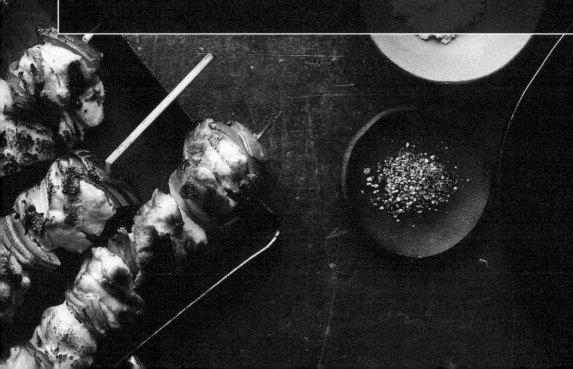

CHAPTER FIVE
DINNER MAINS

One common trend these days is eating the majority of our calories during dinner time. This is where the myth of "eating after 8:00 p.m. makes you gain weight" partially comes from. It's not so much the time of day that matters, but how big your portions are and the quality of your dinner. You should know, however, that eating within 90 minutes of sleeping can negatively impact sleep quality and digestion, which are both factors in your health, so plan and time your dinners wisely. Luckily, the dinners featured here are portioned responsibly while still being satisfying.

FRIED ASIAN-STYLE QUINOA

PREP TIME: 10 MINUTES | COOK TIME: 10 MINUTES | SERVES 4 (SERVING SIZE: 1½ CUPS)
30 MINUTES OR LESS | VEGETARIAN

Peruvian cuisine is all about fusion. This dish is a great representation of what fusion really means, with Peruvian quinoa and Chinese seasonings. Chopped egg is also a common ingredient in Chinese cuisine and adds to the international flair. For an interesting presentation, you can fry the eggs and slide one onto the top of each finished portion.

4 large eggs
¼ teaspoon sea salt
Nonstick cooking spray
1 tablespoon canola oil
1 cup diced celery (about 4 [7-inch] stalks)

1 cup shredded carrots
¼ cup diced red onion
2 tablespoons low-sodium soy sauce
1 cup chopped scallions (green and white parts)
4 cups Basic Quinoa (page 80)

1. Whisk the eggs and salt together in a small bowl.

2. Lightly coat a medium skillet with cooking spray and heat over medium heat. Pour the eggs into the skillet and cook for about 5 minutes, making a rough omelet. Set the skillet aside to cool for 5 minutes, then chop the omelet into 1-inch pieces.

3. Heat the oil in a large skillet over medium heat.

4. Add the celery, carrots, and onion and sauté for 5 minutes or until the vegetables are soft. Stir in the soy sauce.

5. Stir in the scallions, chopped omelet, and quinoa, mixing well.

6. Serve.

CHEF'S NOTE: The vegetables in this recipe are the ones I use most often but feel free to substitute whatever you have on hand.

NUTRITION TIP: Normally this dish is made with white rice but using quinoa instead allows for more fiber and antioxidants.

Per serving: Calories: 376; Total fat: 13g; Sodium: 556mg; Carbohydrates: 51g; Fiber: 10g; Sugar: 7g; Protein: 16g

MOROCCAN-STYLE CHICKPEAS WITH FARRO

PREP TIME: 18 MINUTES | COOK TIME: 18 MINUTES | SERVES 4 (SERVING SIZE: 1½ CUPS)
VEGAN

Don't get intimidated by this recipe because there are a lot of ingredients or you have never used farro before; it is straightforward and fun to make. I made this recipe for a group of friends, and everyone at the table was impressed with the fusion of flavors and interesting texture.

¾ cup dry farro

1 tablespoon extra-virgin olive oil

1 small red onion, diced

2 cups cauliflower florets

1 cup sliced carrots (2 medium carrots)

1 (15-ounce) can chickpeas, drained and rinsed

½ cup low-sodium chicken or vegetable stock

½ teaspoon ground cinnamon

½ teaspoon ground cumin

½ teaspoon ground coriander

½ teaspoon sea salt

1 cup prunes, sliced

½ cup chopped walnuts

1. Cook farro in boiling water as instructed on the package, about 30 minutes. Drain and set aside.

2. Meanwhile, heat the oil in a large saucepan over medium heat. Add the onion, cauliflower, and carrots and sauté for about 3 minutes.

3. Add the chickpeas, stock, cinnamon, cumin, coriander, and salt and bring the mixture to a boil.

4. Reduce the heat to medium low, cover, and simmer for 8 minutes.

5. Stir in the prunes, walnuts, and farro and cook uncovered for another minute, mixing well.

6. Serve.

CHEF'S NOTE: Refrigerate leftovers up to 5 days.

NUTRITION TIP: You can add more protein such as cooked chicken or pork.

Per serving: Calories: 510; Total fat: 17g; Sodium: 451mg; Carbohydrates: 82g; Fiber: 15g; Sugar: 23g; Protein: 16g

SPAGHETTI WITH SPINACH QUESO FRESCO SAUCE

PREP TIME: 10 MINUTES | COOK TIME: 15 MINUTES | SERVES 4 (SERVING SIZE: 1½ CUPS)
30 MINUTES OR LESS | VEGETARIAN

This is a Peruvian-style sauce for pasta that will remind you of pesto with its fresh herbs, garlic, and nuts. Growing up, this was a staple in my household that my mom used to make. As I said before, Peruvian cuisine is all about fusion! This one has an Italian twist.

1 pound whole-grain plus protein spaghetti
1 tablespoon extra-virgin olive oil
¼ cup diced red onion
1 teaspoon minced garlic
5 cups fresh spinach leaves, packed
1 cup fresh basil leaves, packed

¾ cup whole milk (or milk of choice)
10 ounces queso fresco (about 2 cups)
¼ cup chopped walnuts
½ teaspoon sea salt
½ teaspoon freshly ground black pepper

1. Place a large pot of water with a pinch of salt over high heat and bring to a boil. Add the pasta and cook until al dente following the package instructions, about 10 minutes. Drain the pasta and set aside.

2. While the pasta is boiling, heat the oil in a large skillet over medium heat. Add the onion and sauté until translucent, about 3 minutes. Stir in the garlic and sauté 1 minute more, until fragrant.

3. Stir in the spinach and basil and sauté until wilted, about 5 minutes.

4. Transfer the spinach mixture to a blender or food processor. Add the milk, queso fresco, walnuts, salt, and pepper and blend until smooth and creamy.

5. Put the spaghetti back in the pot and add the sauce, mix well, and serve.

> **CHEF'S NOTE:** If you can't find queso fresco, substitute it with feta. Both kinds of cheese are salty, so you don't need to add a lot of salt to this recipe. This pasta goes well with lean beef meatballs (see page 73).

Per serving: Calories: 729; Total fat: 34g; Sodium: 794mg; Carbohydrates: 82g; Fiber: 10g; Sugar: 7g; Protein: 39g

ZUCCHINI CHEESE LASAGNA

PREP TIME: 25 MINUTES | COOK TIME: 40 MINUTES
SERVES 4 (SERVING SIZE: 1 (4-INCH BY 4½-INCH) SLICE)
VEGETARIAN

If you are a fan of cheesy dishes, this is the recipe for you. It doubles up in cheese featuring creamy ricotta and a tempting melted mozzarella topping. Thinly sliced eggplant would also be an excellent addition to these easy layers. This is a great make-ahead dish that refrigerates nicely.

3 cups ricotta cheese
½ cup whole milk (or milk of choice)
1 tablespoon cornstarch
½ teaspoon sea salt

¼ teaspoon freshly ground black pepper
Nonstick cooking spray
3 (8-inch) zucchini, sliced
  lengthwise into long strips
2 ounces shredded mozzarella

1. Preheat oven to 350°F.

2. In a medium bowl, stir together the ricotta, milk, cornstarch, salt, and pepper until well blended. Set aside.

3. Coat a 9-by-13-inch baking dish with cooking spray. Lay a third of the zucchini strips in the dish and spread with a third of the ricotta mixture. Repeat this step twice for a total of six layers. Sprinkle with the mozzarella and cover the dish with aluminum foil.

4. Bake for 30 minutes, then remove the foil and bake for an additional 10 minutes.

5. Serve.

CHEF'S NOTE: Refrigerate leftovers up to 5 days.

NUTRITION TIP: Lasagna normally is made with noodles but substituting with zucchini is another great way to increase your vegetable intake deliciously.

Per serving: Calories: 391; Total fat: 27g; Sodium: 523mg; Carbohydrates: 14g; Fiber: 2g; Sugar: 4g; Protein: 25g

OVEN-BAKED SOLE PACKETS

PREP TIME: 10 MINUTES | COOK TIME: 20 MINUTES | SERVES 4 (SERVING SIZE: 6 OUNCES)
30 MINUTES OR LESS

When cooked in sealed foil or parchment packets, the fish steams with the wine and herbs to create an aromatic, flavorful dish good enough for company. Take care when opening the foil because the escaping steam can burn.

1 cup white wine
½ cup freshly squeezed lemon juice
2 tablespoons extra-virgin olive oil
¼ cup chopped fresh parsley

2 teaspoons sea salt
½ teaspoon freshly ground black pepper
2 pounds sole (or white fish of choice), skinless and boneless, cut into 4 fillets

1. Preheat oven to 400°F. Cut 4 (10-inch) squares of aluminum foil and 4 (10-inch) squares of parchment paper. Place the foil squares on a baking sheet, leaving about 1 inch of space between them. Top each piece of foil with a square of parchment paper and set aside.

2. In a medium bowl, whisk together the wine, lemon juice, extra-virgin olive oil, parsley, salt, and pepper.

3. Place one fish fillet onto each of the parchment squares. Gently pull up the sides of the foil to create a bowl around each piece of fish.

4. Evenly divide the wine mixture among the fish packets and gently pull the edges of each foil packet to the center to form a seal.

5. Bake the fish for 15 minutes or to desired doneness.

6. Transfer fish and sauce into separate bowls and eat immediately.

CHEF'S NOTE: When protein cooks, it shrinks. Each person gets 8 ounces of raw fish, which shrinks to about 6 ounces of cooked fish.

NUTRITION TIP: Baked fish is a lean, protein-rich meal, perfect when accompanied by a fresh salad or Basic Roasted Vegetables (see page 81).

Per serving: Calories: 316; Total fat: 9g; Sodium: 1,397mg; Carbohydrates: 4g; Fiber: <1g; Sugar: 1g; Protein: 42g

SHEET PAN LEMON SALMON WITH ZUCCHINI

PREP TIME: 10 MINUTES | COOK TIME: 12 MINUTES | SERVES 2
(SERVING SIZE: 6 OUNCES SALMON, ⅓ OF THE ZUCCHINI)
30 MINUTES OR LESS | ONE POT

When you're choosing ingredients for a one-baking-sheet preparation, it is best to make sure that they cook for roughly the same amount of time. In this case, zucchini works great because it cooks as fast as salmon. You could also use bell peppers or asparagus with good results, but a vegetable like potatoes will not be successful.

Nonstick cooking spray
1 pound whole salmon fillet, skin on
¾ teaspoon sea salt, divided
¼ teaspoon freshly ground black pepper

¼ teaspoon garlic powder
1 lemon, sliced
3 (7-inch) zucchini, cut lengthwise

1. Preheat oven to 400°F. Cover a 17¼-by-11½-inch rimmed baking sheet with aluminum foil and coat with cooking spray.

2. Place salmon skin-side down on half of the baking sheet. Sprinkle with ½ teaspoon of salt, the pepper, and garlic powder. Top the fish evenly with the lemon slices.

3. Place the zucchini on the other half of the baking sheet and sprinkle with the remaining ¼ teaspoon of salt.

4. Bake for 12 minutes or until the fish flakes when pressed with a fork.

5. Serve.

CHEF'S NOTE: Refrigerate leftovers for up to 2 days.

NUTRITION TIP: Salmon is a good sources of omega-3s, which are heart healthy fats.

Per serving: Calories: 423; Total fat: 21g; Sodium: 1,014mg; Carbohydrates: 17g; Fiber: 6g; Sugar: 5g; Protein: 51g

CALIFORNIA-STYLE STUFFED BELL PEPPERS

PREP TIME: 15 MINUTES | COOK TIME: 55 MINUTES | SERVES 6 (SERVING SIZE: 1 STUFFED BELL PEPPER)

As a spokesperson for several food commodities, one of my jobs is to create recipes. I created this one for the California Avocado Commission. They were generous enough to allow me to share it with you, which is great because it's one of my favorites. I love using California avocados because they're locally grown, fresh, and they taste delicious. The season for this fruit is from March to the end of summer.

1 tablespoon extra-virgin olive oil
½ cup red onion, chopped
1 tablespoon minced garlic
2 (6-inch) celery stalks, diced
1 (6-inch) carrot, diced
1 (6-inch) zucchini, diced

1 pound ground chicken
¼ teaspoon sea salt
⅛ teaspoon freshly ground black pepper
1 cup cherry tomatoes, halved
2 ripe avocados, pitted, peeled, and diced
6 large colorful bell peppers,
   tops cut off and seeded

1. Preheat oven to 350°F.

2. Line a 9-by-13-inch baking dish with aluminum foil and set aside.

3. Heat the oil in a large skillet over medium heat. Add the onion and garlic and sauté for 2 minutes.

4. Add the celery, carrot, and zucchini and sauté for 3 minutes.

5. Stir in the ground chicken and sauté until cooked through, about 6 minutes. Season with the salt and pepper.

6. Remove the skillet from the heat and stir in the cherry tomatoes and avocados.

7. Evenly divide the ground chicken mixture among the bell peppers. Arrange the bell peppers in the prepared baking dish and cover with foil.

8. Bake for 30 minutes.

9. Remove dish from oven and carefully remove the foil. Place back in oven and cook for another 10 minutes or until the peppers are tender.

10. Serve.

CHEF'S NOTE: Large avocados are recommended for this recipe. A large avocado averages about 8 ounces in weight. If using smaller or larger sizes, adjust the quantities accordingly.

NUTRITION TIP: This dish gives you at least two servings of vegetables per day, so it definitely helps you add more plants to your diet.

Per serving: Calories: 362; Total fat: 23g; Sodium: 217mg; Carbohydrates: 24g; Fiber: 10g; Sugar: 7g; Protein: 20g

ROASTED CHICKEN BREAST

PREP TIME: 10 MINUTES | COOK TIME: 12 MINUTES | SERVES 4 (SERVING SIZE: 1 CHICKEN BREAST)
5 INGREDIENTS | 30 MINUTES OR LESS | ONE POT

Roasting is a fast cooking method that can help keep chicken breasts juicy and healthy with little added oil. You have to be aware of your time to ensure the poultry doesn't overcook, so make sure you don't forget your chicken is in the oven. Use a timer!

Nonstick cooking spray
4 boneless skinless chicken breasts

1 teaspoon sea salt
½ teaspoon freshly ground black pepper

1. Preheat oven to 500°F.

2. Coat a 9-by-13-inch baking dish (or a large roasting pan) with cooking spray.

3. Butterfly the chicken on a cutting board. Do this by placing your hand on top of the breast and using a chef's knife to slice into one side of the breast, starting at the thicker end and ending at the thin point. Be careful not to cut all the way through to the other side.

4. Place the chicken breasts with the sides folded out like a butterfly in a single layer in the prepared baking dish. Coat the chicken with more cooking spray and season with the salt and pepper.

5. Bake the chicken for 12 minutes or until the internal temperature is 165°F. Remove from oven and let sit for 5 minutes. The internal temperature of the breasts should be 165°F.

6. Serve.

CHEF'S NOTE: Cooled roasted chicken can be stored in an airtight container in the refrigerator for up to 5 days.

NUTRITION TIP: This cooked chicken can be used as a protein in the grain bowl and salad recipes in this book.

Per serving: Calories: 111; Total fat: 3g; Sodium: 762mg; Carbohydrates: <1g; Fiber: <1g; Sugar: 0g; Protein: 23g

SHEET PAN OREGANO CHICKEN WITH BUTTERNUT SQUASH

PREP TIME: 10 MINUTES | COOK TIME: 14 MINUTES
SERVES 4 (SERVING SIZE: 6 OUNCES OF CHICKEN, 3 OUNCES OF BUTTERNUT SQUASH)
30 MINUTES OR LESS

Baking sheet recipes are a great meal because there's not a lot of cleanup and everything is cooked all at once! Cook once and eat twice by packing it for lunch the next day.

Nonstick cooking spray

2 pounds boneless skinless chicken breasts, butterflied (see page 63)

1 tablespoon dried oregano

2 teaspoons freshly squeezed lemon juice

¾ teaspoon sea salt, divided

¼ teaspoon freshly ground black pepper

1 pound butternut squash, peeled, seeded, and cubed

¼ teaspoon garlic powder

1. Preheat oven to 450°F.

2. Cover a 17¼-by-11½-inch rimmed baking sheet with aluminum foil and coat with cooking spray.

3. Place the chicken in a single layer on one side of the baking sheet.

4. In a small bowl, stir together the oregano, lemon juice, ½ teaspoon of salt, and the pepper. Drizzle the mixture over the chicken.

5. Arrange the butternut squash in a single layer on the other side of the baking sheet and season with the remaining ¼ teaspoon of salt, a pinch of black pepper, and the garlic powder.

6. Coat the chicken and butternut squash with cooking spray.

7. Bake for 14 minutes or until the internal temperature of the chicken is 165°F.

8. Serve.

CHEF'S NOTE: Since oven temperatures vary, use a meat thermometer to make sure the chicken is done. To freeze the cooked chicken, let cool and seal in plastic freezer bags in individual portions, squeezing out as much air as possible. They can be stored for up to 3 months.

Per serving: Calories: 271; Total fat: 5g; Sodium: 802mg; Carbohydrates: 13g; Fiber: 4g; Sugar: 2g; Protein: 47g

GRILLED YOGURT CHICKEN SKEWERS

PREP TIME: 20 MINUTES | COOK TIME: 20 MINUTES
SERVES 4 (SERVING SIZE: 4 SKEWERS WITH ABOUT 4 OUNCES OF CHICKEN, 3 TO 4 ONION CHUNKS)
ONE POT

This recipe takes me to the islands of Greece, where they often cook with yogurt. It is commonly used in dips, marinades, and salads in this region.

1 large red onion

2 (16-ounce) containers 2% plain Greek yogurt

2 teaspoons sea salt

¼ teaspoon freshly ground black pepper

3 pounds boneless skinless chicken thighs, cut into 1-inch cubes

2 medium red onions, cut into 1-inch chunks

1. In a food processor, grind the large onion.

2. In a large bowl, stir together the processed onion, yogurt, salt, and pepper until well blended.

3. Add the chicken to the bowl, stirring to make sure the poultry is completely coated in the yogurt mixture. Cover with plastic wrap and let sit for 20 minutes.

4. Preheat the grill to 400°F.

5. Thread the chicken and onion chunks onto wooden skewers.

6. Cook for 20 minutes on the grill, turning every 4 minutes.

CHEF'S NOTE: If you don't have a grill, you can use the oven (preheat to 450°F). Place the skewers over a sheet pan using a grill rack on top. Bake for 10 minutes on each side.

NUTRITION TIP: Yogurt is the perfect poultry marinade because the calcium and lactic acid in this creamy dairy product very gently break down the protein in the chicken. This creates a tender and juicy finished dish.

Per serving: Calories: 596; Total fat: 26g; Sodium: 1,751mg; Carbohydrates: 17g; Fiber: 2g; Sugar: 13g; Protein: 71g

PRIMAVERA FUSILLI WITH CHICKEN SAUSAGE

PREP TIME: 10 MINUTES | COOK TIME: 15 MINUTES | SERVES 4 (SERVING SIZE: 2½ CUPS)
30 MINUTES OR LESS

This is a wonderfully simple meal to prepare for a special occasion or just for yourself. It contains all you need for a healthy lifestyle such as protein, carbohydrates, fats, and vegetables. Leftovers heat up nicely the next day, so you won't have to worry about planning your lunch.

1 pound whole-grain plus protein fusilli

1 tablespoon extra-virgin olive oil

4 cooked chicken sausages,
   cut into ½-inch slices

¼ red onion, diced

1 (7-inch) zucchini, cut into ½-inch slices

½ cup shredded carrots

1 teaspoon sea salt

1 cup cherry tomatoes, halved

¼ cup chopped fresh basil

1. Bring a large pot of water to a boil. Cook pasta according to package instructions, until al dente, about 10 minutes. Drain and set aside.

2. While the pasta is cooking, heat the oil in a large skillet over medium heat. Add the sausages and onion and sauté for about 3 minutes, until the onion is translucent.

3. Add the zucchini, carrots, and salt and sauté for 8 to 10 minutes, or until the vegetables are softened and the sausage is browned.

4. Stir in the cherry tomatoes and basil and cook for another 1 to 2 minutes.

5. Add the pasta to the sausage and vegetable mixture and toss to combine.

6. Serve.

CHEF'S NOTE: I love using pasta with higher protein amounts. Usually these kinds of pasta are made with chickpea or quinoa flour in addition to semolina.

NUTRITION TIP: You can add more vegetables or substitute with ones you enjoy.

Per serving: Calories: 595; Total fat: 19g; Sodium: 1,220mg; Carbohydrates: 83g; Fiber: 10g; Sugar: 7g; Protein: 35g

CHICKEN VEGETABLE STEW

PREP TIME: 10 MINUTES | COOK TIME: 1 HOUR | SERVES 3 (SERVING SIZE: 2⅓ CUPS)
ONE POT

Almost every kitchen in Peru has a special seasoning called Ajinomoto in their pantry, which is a brand of MSG (monosodium glutamate). Unfortunately, this ingredient has gotten a bad reputation from flawed and inaccurate studies even though there is no conclusive research that shows an association between MSG consumption and adverse reactions. The International Headache Society removed MSG from its list of headache triggers because of the lack of proof. To learn more about the myth of MSG, visit my blog and view the article titled "Debunking the Myth Behind MSG."

1 tablespoon extra-virgin olive oil
½ cup diced red onion
1 whole chicken, skinned and cut into 10 pieces
1 (14½-ounce) can no-salt-added tomato sauce
1 (14½-ounce) can no-salt-added diced tomatoes

½ teaspoon sea salt
1 teaspoon MSG
1 teaspoon ground cumin
2 cups mixed frozen vegetables (corn, green beans, carrots)

1. Heat the oil in a large stockpot over medium heat. Add the onion and sauté for about 3 minutes, until the onion is translucent.

2. Add the chicken, tomato sauce, diced tomatoes, salt, MSG, and cumin and bring to a boil.

3. Reduce the heat to medium low, cover, and simmer for 10 minutes.

4. Stir in the frozen vegetables and continue simmering for 35 minutes, stirring occasionally.

5. Uncover and cook for 10 more minutes over low heat, or until the internal temperature of the chicken is 165°F.

6. Serve.

> **CHEF'S NOTE:** You can add any frozen vegetable to this delicious, easy-to-make stew.
>
> **NUTRITION TIP:** MSG has two-thirds less sodium than table salt and can enhance the flavors of food while decreasing the need for salt. It works really well in a savory recipe because MSG is umami.

Per serving: Calories: 447; Total fat: 12g; Sodium: 1,321mg; Carbohydrates: 29g; Fiber: 6g; Sugar: 16g; Protein: 58g

SHEET PAN THIN PIZZA WITH CANADIAN BACON

PREP TIME: 5 MINUTES | COOK TIME: 6 MINUTES | SERVES 2 (SERVING SIZE: 1 PIZZA)
30 MINUTES OR LESS | ONE POT

Who doesn't like pizza? Pizza is one of my favorite foods. I love it so much that I created a guilt-free version, and I make it almost weekly. I'm pleased to share my pizza recipe with you, including simple but delectable toppings that work for any meal, including breakfast.

2 (10-by-8-inch) slices whole-grain lavash
½ cup pizza sauce
6 ounces shredded mozzarella

6 ounces cooked Canadian bacon, chopped
1 red bell pepper, seeded and thinly sliced
½ small red onion, thinly sliced

1. Preheat oven to 350°F.

2. Cover a 17¼-by-11½-inch rimmed baking sheet with aluminum foil and coat with cooking spray.

3. Place the lavash on the prepared baking sheet and spread each piece with half the pizza sauce, about ½ inch from the sides.

4. Top the sauce with the mozzarella, bacon, bell pepper, and onion.

5. Bake the pizza for 6 minutes or until the cheese is melted.

6. Serve.

> **CHEF'S NOTE:** You can eat the second pizza for breakfast.
>
> **NUTRITION TIP:** I substituted thin lavash bread for pizza dough to lower the carbohydrates amount in this recipe.

Per serving: Calories: 433; Total fat: 15g; Sodium: 1,837mg; Carbohydrates: 36g; Fiber: 4g; Sugar: 7g; Protein: 33g

ROASTED PORK WITH CILANTRO SAUCE

PREP TIME: 10 MINUTES | COOK TIME: 40 MINUTES | SERVES 4 (SERVING SIZE: 6 OUNCES OF PORK PLUS 2 TO 3 TABLESPOONS SAUCE)

One of the keys to culinary success and a healthy lifestyle is meal planning. If you make this recipe at the beginning of the week, you'll have delicious protein ready to add to salads, soups, or bowls. Visit my blog to see a video on how to make this recipe.

For the pork

Nonstick cooking spray

2 pounds pork loin

Sea salt

¼ teaspoon ground black pepper

¼ teaspoon ground cumin

¼ teaspoon garlic powder

For the cilantro sauce

1½ teaspoons extra-virgin olive oil

1 small onion, quartered

1 tablespoon chili paste

1 teaspoon minced garlic

½ cup fresh cilantro, chopped

2 tablespoons water

To make the pork

1. Preheat oven to 375°F.

2. Cover a baking sheet with aluminum foil and coat with cooking spray.

3. Place the pork on a cutting board.

4. In a small bowl, combine the salt, pepper, cumin, and garlic powder until well mixed and rub each side of the pork with the spices, making sure to cover the entire surface.

5. Place the pork on the prepared baking sheet and roast for about 40 minutes or until the internal temperature of the pork is 145°F. Let rest for 10 minutes and slice.

To make the cilantro sauce

1. Heat a medium skillet over medium-high heat for 2 minutes. Place the oil, onion, chili paste, and garlic in the skillet and sauté for about 3 minutes.

2. Transfer the onion mixture to a blender along with the cilantro and water. Blend until it is a smooth consistency. Serve the cilantro sauce on top of the sliced pork.

Per serving: Calories: 364; Total fat: 18g; Sodium: 848mg; Carbohydrates: 6g; Fiber: 1g; Sugar: 2g; Protein: 43g

SHEET PAN MARINATED ASIAN PORK LOIN WITH CARROTS AND ONIONS

PREP TIME: 15 MINUTES, PLUS 1 HOUR TO MARINATE | COOK TIME: 14 MINUTES | SERVES 4 (SERVING SIZE: 6 OUNCES OF PORK, 1 CARROT, ¼ RED ONION)

This is one of my favorite baking sheet recipes, and I make it often. Lean cuts of pork don't have a lot of fat and taste mild, so they need a little help in the flavor department. Marinating pork in these seasonings enhances the flavors of this healthy, lean protein.

For the marinade

⅓ cup low-sodium soy sauce

1 tablespoon canola oil

1 tablespoon brown sugar

1 teaspoon minced garlic

½ teaspoon sea salt

¼ teaspoon freshly ground black pepper

For the pork

1½ pounds boneless, center-cut pork loin chops

Nonstick cooking spray

4 carrots, peeled and cut into 1-inch slices

1 red onion, cut into 1- to 2-inch chunks

¼ teaspoon garlic powder

Extra-virgin olive oil spray

4 scallions, sliced (green and white parts)

To make the marinade

1. Whisk together the soy sauce, oil, brown sugar, garlic, salt, and pepper until well blended and pour the marinade into a large sealable plastic bag.

2. Add the pork and seal the bag, squeezing out as much air as possible. Let the pork marinate for at least 1 hour at room temperature, or overnight in the refrigerator.

To make the pork

1. Preheat oven to 450°F.

2. Cover a 17¼-by-11½-inch rimmed baking sheet with aluminum foil and coat with cooking spray.

3. Place the pork on the prepared baking sheet and discard the marinade. Arrange the carrots and onions around the pork.

4. Sprinkle the vegetables with the garlic powder and coat the pork and vegetables with extra-virgin olive oil spray.

5. Bake for 14 minutes or until the internal temperature of the pork is 145°F.

6. Top with scallions and serve.

CHEF'S NOTE: The longer the pork marinates, the better it will taste. Consider starting this meal preparation the night before for best results.

Per serving: Calories: 289; Total fat: 10g; Sodium: 1,371mg; Carbohydrates: 15g; Fiber: 3g; Sugar: 7g; Protein: 37g

MANGO PULLED PORK WITH BELL PEPPERS

PREP TIME: 10 MINUTES | COOK TIME: 45 MINUTES | SERVES 6 (SERVING SIZE: 1½ CUPS)
ONE POT

I love this recipe because it has multiple culinary uses. Once the pork is prepared, you can mix it with your favorite pasta, use it to fill a baked sweet potato, or for your Taco Tuesdays. I actually have a video on my blog outlining the versatility of this recipe. Visit ManuelVillacorta.com to watch the video.

4 pounds pork loin, cut into 3-inch cubes
3 bell peppers (any color), roughly chopped
2 jalapeño peppers, seeded and diced
1 medium red onion, roughly chopped
1 mango, peeled, pitted, and chopped

¼ cup red wine vinegar
1 tablespoon minced garlic
Sea salt
Freshly ground black pepper
½ cup fresh cilantro, chopped

1. Put all the ingredients in an Instant Pot®. Make sure to mix all ingredients well, so everything gets coated with the sauce.

2. Cook on "Manual" for 45 minutes.

3. When done, turn the pressure valve to release the pressure and open the lid.

4. Drain the liquid by putting the pork and bell peppers in a colander.

5. Place the pork mixture onto a cutting board and shred with two forks.

6. Put the shredded pork mixture in a bowl. Mix in the cilantro and serve.

> **NUTRITION TIP:** Originally, this recipe was made with barbecue sauce. I used mango instead because it has natural sugars, is nutrient-dense, and is very high in vitamins and minerals.

Per serving: Calories: 484; Total fat: 22g; Sodium: 1,072mg; Carbohydrates: 15g; Fiber: 2g; Sugar: 7g; Protein: 58g

LEAN BEEF MEATBALLS

PREP TIME: 10 MINUTES | COOK TIME: 25 MINUTES | SERVES 6 (SERVING SIZE: 4 MEATBALLS)

Every Italian home has their own way to make a meatball. I've gained inspiration on how to create meatballs over the years by watching my Italian friends. I made this recipe based on their stories, putting my own twist on it. You can also make your mark by changing the herbs to suit your own palate.

Nonstick cooking spray
2 pounds 93% lean ground beef
½ cup whole milk (or milk of choice)
2 large eggs, lightly beaten
2 ounces shredded Parmesan

1 tablespoon dried oregano
1 tablespoon dried basil
1 teaspoon minced garlic
1 teaspoon sea salt
½ teaspoon freshly ground black pepper

1. Preheat oven to 400°F.

2. Line a baking sheet with aluminum foil and coat with cooking spray.

3. In a large bowl, combine the beef, milk, eggs, Parmesan, oregano, basil, garlic, salt, and pepper. Use your hands to mix the ingredients together, making sure they are well distributed.

4. Scoop the meat mixture up using a ⅓-cup measure and roll it into 2-inch meatballs with wet hands. Place the meatballs on the prepared baking sheet.

5. Bake for 25 minutes or until the internal temperature of the meatballs is 160°F.

6. Remove the meatballs from oven and let sit for a few minutes before serving.

> **CHEF'S NOTE:** These meatballs are juicy and their lightly herbed flavor goes well with many dishes. Eat them with your marinara sauce of choice, pasta, pesto, or quinoa. You can even cut them into pieces and serve as little appetizers. Alternatively, enjoy them with your favorite salad.
>
> **NUTRITION TIP:** Substituting 80% lean for 93% lean beef will reduce the amount of saturated fat in this recipe.

Per serving: Calories: 295; Total fat: 16g; Sodium: 696mg; Carbohydrates: 3g; Fiber: 2g; Sugar: 1g; Protein: 36g

POLENTA WITH GROUND BEEF CASSEROLE

PREP TIME: 25 MINUTES | COOK TIME: 1 HOUR 15 MINUTES | SERVES 4
(SERVING SIZE: 1 [4-INCH BY 4½-INCH] SLICE)

Polenta is cornmeal commonly found in Italian cuisine. Polenta can be prepared from scratch to produce creamy dishes, but in this recipe, I used cooked plain polenta for convenience. This is a perfect meal to cook over the weekend to be enjoyed during the week ahead.

Nonstick cooking spray
1 tablespoon extra-virgin olive oil
1 small red onion, diced
1 tablespoon minced garlic
2 pounds 93% lean ground beef
2 (14.5-ounce) cans no-salt-added
   tomato sauce

1 (14½-ounce) can no-salt-added
   diced tomatoes
1 tablespoon dried oregano
½ teaspoon sea salt
¼ teaspoon freshly ground black pepper
2 (18-ounce) cooked polenta tubes,
   cut into ½-inch slices
2 ounces shredded mozzarella cheese

1. Preheat oven to 350°F.

2. Coat a 9-by-13-inch baking dish with cooking spray.

3. Heat the oil in a large skillet over medium heat.

4. Add the onion and sauté for 3 minutes, until translucent. Add the garlic and cook for another minute, until fragrant.

5. Stir in the ground beef and sauté for 7 to 8 minutes or until the meat is no longer pink.

6. Stir in the tomato sauce, diced tomatoes, oregano, salt, and pepper and simmer over medium-low heat for 15 minutes.

7. Layer the casserole in the prepared dish as follows: a third of the polenta slices, then a third of the sauce. Repeat the process twice for a total of 6 layers. Top with mozzarella and cover the dish with aluminum foil. Bake for 40 minutes.

8. Remove the foil and bake for another 10 minutes.

9. Serve.

CHEF'S NOTE: Refrigerate leftovers up to 5 days.

NUTRITION TIP: The canning process for tomatoes makes lycopene, an antioxidant, more bioavailable. This means the body can absorb more lycopene from canned than from fresh tomatoes.

Per serving: Calories: 636; Total fat: 21g; Sodium: 1,353mg; Carbohydrates: 60g; Fiber: 8g; Sugar: 18g; Protein: 56g

BEEF VEGETABLE STIR-FRY

PREP TIME: 10 MINUTES | COOK TIME: 10 MINUTES | SERVES 4 (SERVING SIZE: 2 CUPS)
30 MINUTES OR LESS | ONE POT

Stir-frys are a wild-card recipe to make during a busy week because depending on the number of ingredients, this dish can take longer than you want to spend in the kitchen. I often prepare one for dinner using simple ingredients if I'm pressed for time but want something really satisfying. This one can be prepared in 10 minutes!

1 tablespoon canola oil
1 small red onion, chopped
1 red bell pepper, chopped
1 yellow bell pepper, chopped
1 orange bell pepper, chopped

2 (7-inch) celery stalks, sliced
1 pound sirloin steak, cut into strips
1 teaspoon sea salt
¼ teaspoon freshly ground black pepper
¼ cup fresh parsley, chopped

1. Heat the oil in a large skillet over medium heat. Add the onion, bell peppers, and celery and sauté for 5 minutes, or until the vegetables soften. Remove the veggies from the skillet and set aside in a small bowl.

2. Add the beef, salt, and pepper to the skillet and sauté for 5 to 7 minutes or until the beef is fully cooked.

3. Add the vegetables back to the skillet and stir.

4. Top with the parsley and serve.

> **NUTRITION TIP:** All peppers are loaded with antioxidants. The variation in color is due to the level of carotenoids they contain.

Per serving: Calories: 310; Total fat: 20g; Sodium: 664mg; Carbohydrates: 9g; Fiber: 3g; Sugar: 4g; Protein: 23g

EGGPLANT CHICKPEA BEEF STEW

PREP TIME: 5 MINUTES | COOK TIME: 50 MINUTES | SERVES 4 (SERVING SIZE: 2 CUPS)

This is a recipe inspired by my mother, who is Arab in origin. On one of her trips to San Francisco from Lima, Peru, she made this delicious recipe for me. I'm sharing it with you because sometimes humble ingredients combine in an unexpectedly spectacular manner. Enjoy!

1 tablespoon extra-virgin olive oil

2 medium eggplants, cut into 2-inch pieces

1 red onion, sliced

2 pounds beef stew, cubed

2 (15-ounce) cans chickpeas, drained and rinsed

1 (6-ounce) can no-salt-added tomato paste

¼ cup water

1 tablespoon garlic, minced

2 teaspoons sea salt

½ teaspoon freshly ground black pepper

½ teaspoon ground cumin

1. Heat the oil in a large skillet over medium heat. Add the eggplants and onion and sauté for about 4 minutes, until softened. Transfer the vegetables to an Instant Pot®.

2. Add the beef, chickpeas, tomato paste, water, garlic, salt, pepper, and cumin and cook on "Manual" high pressure for 40 minutes.

3. When done, turn the pressure valve to release the pressure and open the lid.

4. Serve.

Per serving: Calories: 705; Total fat: 20g; Sodium: 1,340mg; Carbohydrates: 67g; Fiber: 21g; Sugar: 23g; Protein: 67g

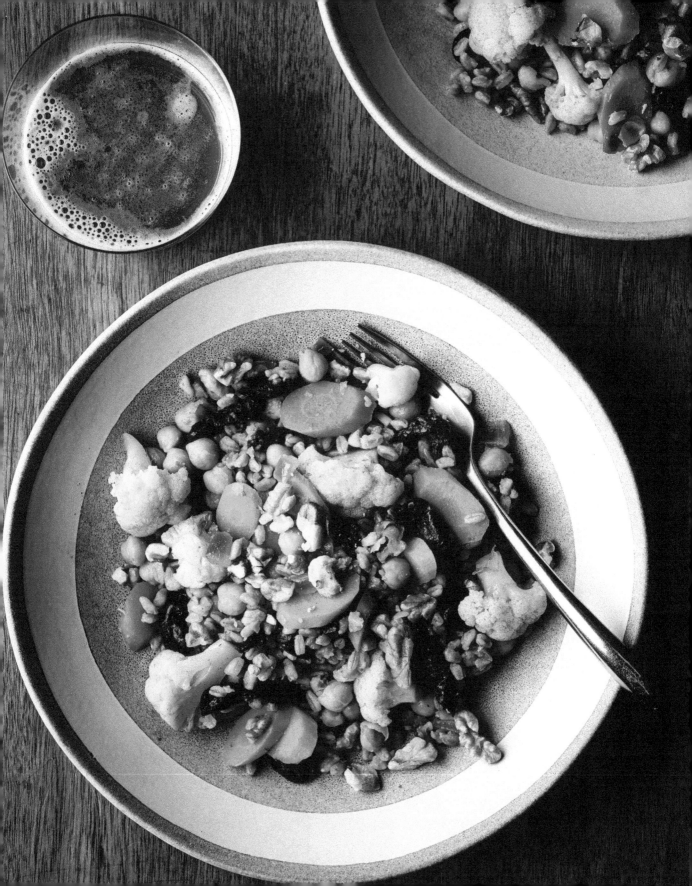

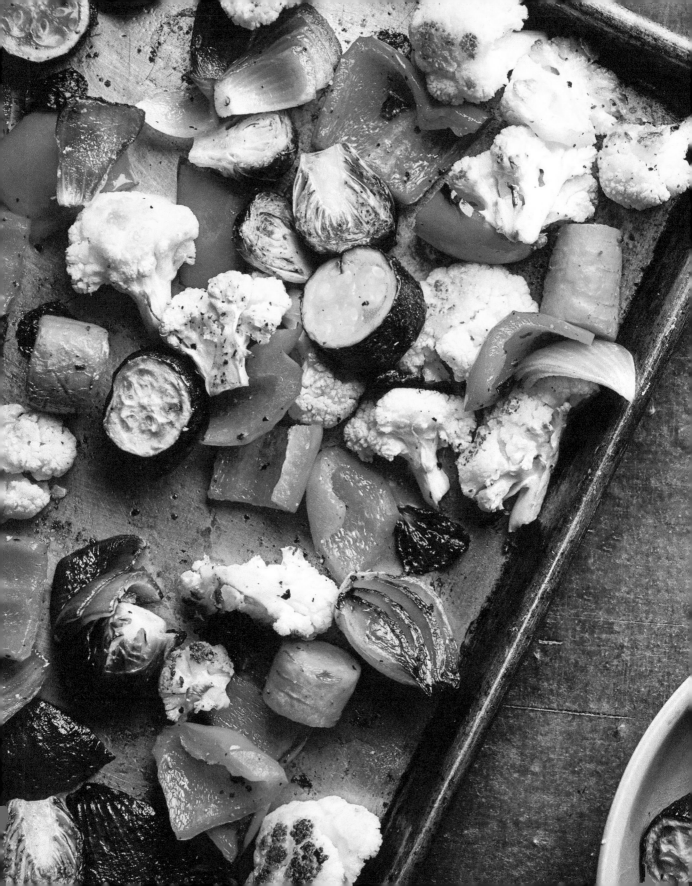

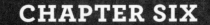

CHAPTER SIX

BASIC SIDES

This section contains "sides essentials" so to speak in that they are super simple in execution, but you can almost guarantee you'll be cooking them nonstop once you get started. That's because these basic sides can be added to many other recipes in need of a healthy grain, starch, or veggie for a balanced meal. Once you've mastered the ability to whip up these delicious sides, the frequent question— "What should I make with this?"—will always have an answer.

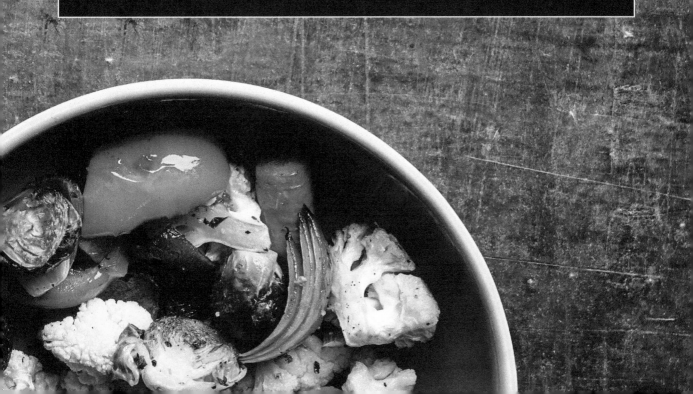

BASIC QUINOA

PREP TIME: 5 MINUTES | COOK TIME: 20 MINUTES | SERVES 3 (SERVING SIZE: 1 CUP)
5 INGREDIENTS | 30 MINUTES OR LESS | ONE POT | VEGAN

Just like Italians prefer pasta that is al dente, I'm a Peruvian who likes my quinoa al dente. To add that extra bite, I use a little less water than traditional preparations. If you want more tender quinoa, use 2 cups of water instead.

1 cup white quinoa

1¾ cups water or low-sodium
  chicken or vegetable broth

½ teaspoon sea salt

1. Place the quinoa in a sieve and rinse under cold water until the water runs clear. Transfer it to a medium saucepan and add the water and salt.

2. Bring to a boil over medium-high heat, cover, and reduce the heat to low. Simmer until all of the water has been absorbed, 15 to 20 minutes.

3. Fluff the quinoa with a fork and serve.

> **CHEF'S NOTE:** Quinoa will keep in the refrigerator for 3 to 5 days.

Per serving: Calories: 128; Total fat: 2g; Sodium: 233mg; Carbohydrates: 22g; Fiber: 2g; Sugar: 0g; Protein: 5g

BASIC ROASTED VEGETABLES

PREP TIME: 15 MINUTES | COOK TIME: 20 MINUTES | SERVES 4 (SERVING SIZE: 2 CUPS)
ONE POT | VEGAN

In my private practice, one of the most common questions I get asked is, "How can I increase my vegetable intake?" I always tell my clients to roast their veggies! It's the easiest way to make tasty and delicious vegetables that last all week. Add them to soups, salads, sandwiches, and more. The options are endless.

1 red onion
1 bell pepper
1 zucchini
1 carrot
1 cup Brussels sprouts

1 head cauliflower
2 tablespoons extra-virgin olive oil
1½ teaspoon sea salt
½ teaspoon freshly ground black pepper

1. Preheat oven to 450°F.

2. Chop the onion, bell pepper, zucchini, carrot, Brussels sprouts, and cauliflower into pieces of equivalent size, about 1 to 2 inches.

3. Place the chopped vegetables in a roasting pan and toss them with the oil, salt, and pepper.

4. Roast the vegetables for 20 minutes, or until they are tender and their edges are browned.

5. Serve.

> **NUTRITION TIP:** Use a rainbow of colors with your vegetables. Different colors mean different antioxidants, each of which has distinctive health benefits.

Per serving: Calories: 139; Total fat: 8g; Sodium: 938mg; Carbohydrates: 17g; Fiber: 7g; Sugar: 7g; Protein: 5g

BASIC INSTANT POT® BLACK BEANS

PREP TIME: 5 MINUTES | COOK TIME: 40 MINUTES | SERVES 4 (SERVING SIZE: 2½ CUPS)
VEGAN

I was sitting with a Peruvian client in my office, and he was complaining that his bean recipe never turned out as delicious as his mother's beans. He couldn't figure out the missing ingredient. I told him to try adding MSG. When he returned, he surprised me with a huge hug and a happy, "OMG, now I'm making beans like my mom!"

1 pound dried black beans
1 small red onion, diced
1 red bell pepper, diced
1 tablespoon minced garlic

½ teaspoon ground cumin
1 teaspoon sea salt
1 teaspoon MSG

1. Pour beans into a large pot and cover with cold water. Bring to a boil over medium-high heat and then simmer for 5 minutes.

2. Drain the beans and discard the water. Pour the beans into an Instant Pot® and add the onion, bell pepper, garlic, cumin, salt, and MSG. Pour water into the Instant Pot® so that the ingredients are covered by a half inch.

3. Cook on "Manual" high pressure for 35 minutes.

4. When done, turn the pressure valve to release the pressure and open the lid.

5. Serve.

> **NUTRITION TIP:** Boiling the beans before putting them in the Instant Pot® makes them more digestible by removing the fiber raffinose. This way, you can enjoy your beans without them causing gas.

Per serving: Calories: 229; Total fat: 1g; Sodium: 517mg; Carbohydrates: 50g; Fiber: 11g; Sugar: 3g; Protein: 16g

BASIC INSTANT POT® BROWN RICE

PREP TIME: 5 MINUTES | COOK TIME: 22 MINUTES | SERVES 4 (SERVING SIZE: 1½ CUPS)
5 INGREDIENTS | 30 MINUTES OR LESS | ONE POT | VEGAN

The trick to creating fast, healthy meals is having the best ingredients on hand. You can't make it if you don't have it! Try to get in the habit of cooking brown rice every week as a staple carbohydrate. This nutty-tasting grain can last in the refrigerator for up to 5 days. I usually make at least 3 cups of rice at a time.

2 cups brown rice
2 cups water

1 teaspoon extra-virgin olive oil
1 teaspoon sea salt

1. Put the rice, water, oil, and salt in an Instant Pot® and mix well.

2. Cook on "Manual" high pressure for 22 minutes.

3. When done, turn the pressure valve to release the pressure and open the lid.

4. Serve.

CHEF'S NOTE: You can easily scale the quantities for this recipe up or down to suit your needs. Just make sure you use 1 cup of water for every 1 cup of rice. To make on the stovetop, it's usually 2 cups of water to 1 cup of rice.

NUTRITION TIP: This side can be used with almost any of your main dishes.

Per serving: Calories: 350; Total fat: 7g; Sodium: 581mg; Carbohydrates: 70g; Fiber: 4g; Sugar: 0g; Protein: 8g

BROWN RICE AND BEAN CROQUETTES

PREP TIME: 10 MINUTES | COOK TIME: 35 MINUTES | SERVES 4 (SERVING SIZE: 2 CROQUETTES)
VEGAN

In Peru, we eat a lot of rice and beans, and we always have leftovers. This is a great recipe to cook with your leftovers. In Peru, we call it Tacu Tacu. The benefit of this pairing is the ingredients are inexpensive, and the combination creates a protein on par nutritionally with meat.

1 tablespoon canola oil
1 large yellow onion, chopped fine
3 cloves garlic, crushed
1 tablespoon aji amarillo paste or
  mild chili paste

1½ cups cooked black beans
2 cups cooked brown rice
Nonstick cooking spray

1. Heat the oil in a large skillet over medium heat. Add the onion and garlic and sauté for 3 to 5 minutes or until soft.

2. Add the aji amarillo paste and beans and gently mash them into the onion mixture using a spatula or a fork.

3. Stir in the rice and continue cooking until a dense mass forms. Turn off the heat and let cool.

4. Preheat oven to 400°F.

5. Lightly coat a baking sheet with cooking spray and set aside.

6. Divide the bean mixture into 8 equal portions. Gently roll each portion with your hands to form an oval and place them on the prepared baking sheet. Coat the tops with cooking spray.

7. Bake until crisp and golden, 20 to 30 minutes.

8. Serve warm.

CHEF'S NOTE: Aji amarillo can be found at any Latino store. If you can't find aji amarillo, you can use any chili paste.

NUTRITION TIP: In Peru, they deep-fry the croquettes, but replacing the frying with baking reduces the amount of oil and fat in this recipe.

Per serving: Calories: 254; Total fat: 6g; Sodium: 48mg; Carbohydrates: 43g; Fiber: 8g; Sugar: 3g; Protein: 9g

ROASTED POTATOES

PREP TIME: 5 MINUTES | COOK TIME: 30 MINUTES | SERVES 4 (SERVING SIZE: 6 OUNCES)
5 INGREDIENTS | VEGAN

Contrary to popular belief, potatoes are a nutritious vegetable. It all depends on how you cook them. Any type of potato, such as buttery fingerlings, tender baby potatoes, and even plain white potatoes, works beautifully.

2 pounds gold potatoes, washed and quartered
1 tablespoon extra-virgin olive oil
½ teaspoon sea salt

¼ teaspoon freshly ground black pepper
1 teaspoon garlic powder

1. Preheat oven to 400°F.

2. Cover a baking sheet with aluminum foil and set aside.

3. In a large bowl, toss the potatoes with the olive oil, salt, pepper, and garlic powder.

4. Spread the potatoes on the prepared baking sheet in a single layer.

5. Bake for 25 to 30 minutes or until the potatoes are tender and lightly browned.

6. Serve.

NUTRITION TIP: Roasting is a more nutritious alternative to frying because you aren't adding fat to the dish.

Per serving: Calories: 189; Total fat: 4g; Sodium: 327mg; Carbohydrates: 36g; Fiber: 6g; Sugar: 2g; Protein: 4g

STEAMED BROCCOLI

PREP TIME: 5 MINUTES | COOK TIME: 10 MINUTES | SERVES 4 (SERVING SIZE: 4 CUPS)
5 INGREDIENTS | 30 MINUTES OR LESS | VEGAN

Steaming vegetables is an easy, quick, and nutritious way to get your vegetable intake for the day. You'll need a steamer, covered pan, or microwaveable bowl.

1 cup water
1 head broccoli, cut into florets
1 teaspoon extra-virgin olive oil

Sea salt
Freshly squeezed lemon juice

1. Pour the water into a 4-quart pot.

2. Place a steamer rack inside the pot.

3. Place the broccoli on top of the rack.

4. Cover the pot and bring the water to boil over medium-high heat (about 4 minutes). Once the water reaches a boil, lower the heat to low and let it simmer for another 4 minutes or longer if you like soft vegetables.

5. Drain the broccoli, transfer to a large bowl, and let them cool for about 5 minutes. Season them with the oil, salt, and lemon juice.

6. Serve.

CHEF'S NOTE: You can use the microwave if you don't want to use the steamer. Wash the broccoli florets and place them in a large bowl. Cover the bowl with a microwaveable cover and microwave for about 7 minutes. This will leave them crunchy yet tender. If you like soft vegetables, cook for another minute or two.

NUTRITION TIP: You can follow the same steps with any other vegetable but be aware that the times of cooking will vary.

Per serving: Calories: 53; Total fat: 2g; Sodium: 41mg; Carbohydrates: 8g; Fiber: 5g; Sugar: 3g; Protein: 5g

BASIC CLASSIC PASTA

PREP TIME: 6 MINUTES | COOK TIME: 10 MINUTES | SERVES 4 (SERVING SIZE: 4 CUPS)
5 INGREDIENTS | 30 MINUTES OR LESS | VEGETARIAN

This is your most basic pasta recipe. I used spaghetti pasta to demonstrate how to cook pasta but you can use any type of pasta (penne, rotini, linguine). Check the cooking times on the box.

1 (14.5-ounce) box spaghetti

1 teaspoon sea salt

1 tablespoon extra-virgin olive oil

1. Bring 4 to 6 quarts of water to boil in a large pot. Add the salt and olive oil.

2. Add pasta.

3. Read the instructions on the box for cooking time. Normally for authentic "al dente" pasta boil for 8 minutes. For tender pasta boil additional 2 minutes.

4. Drain well and serve with your favorite sauce.

NUTRITION TIP: You can season the cooked pasta with another tablespoon of extra-virgin olive oil, sea salt, and black pepper, mix in some Parmesan cheese, and voila! Enjoy.

Per serving: Calories: 411; Total fat: 5g; Sodium: 589mg; Carbohydrates: 77g; Fiber: 3g; Sugar: 3g; Protein: 13g

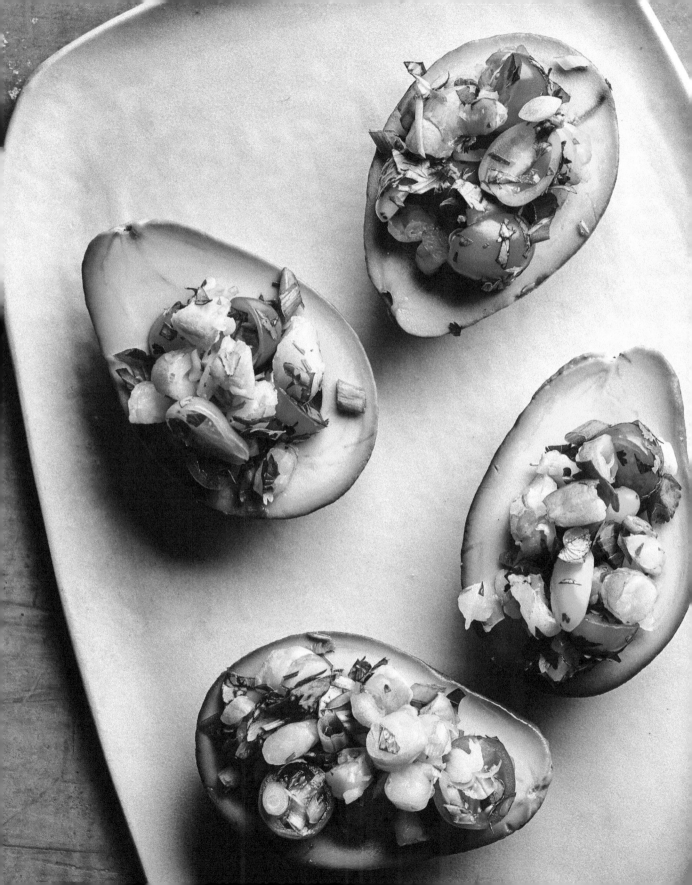

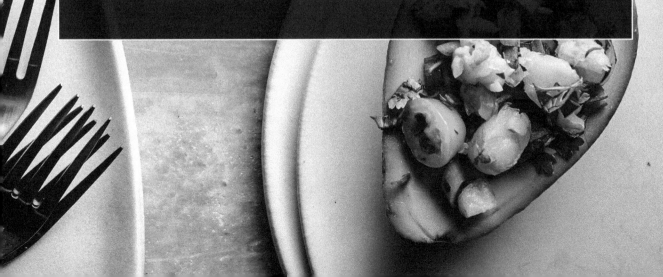

CHAPTER SEVEN

SMART SALADS (AND DRESSINGS)

Salads too often are given short shrift, but they really should be considered the secret stars of a meal. Think about it: By combining just a few (or a lot) of ingredients with the added punch of a fantastic dressing, you bring delightful contrasts to the table. Salads can be cold or warm (yes, really), soft or crunchy, and filled with surprising ingredients. Consider these salad recipes as a way to really show off your culinary skills.

CARAMELIZED ONION WALNUT SALAD

PREP TIME: 5 MINUTES | COOK TIME: 12 MINUTES | SERVES 2 (SERVING SIZE: 2 CUPS)
30 MINUTES OR LESS | ONE POT | VEGAN

When I moved to the United States 30 years ago, I ate cold salads regularly. Somehow, I developed an aversion to cold foods after that. But knowing that salads were good for me and packed with nutrition, I started being creative and making warm salads. Here's one of my favorites.

2 tablespoons extra-virgin olive oil
1 red onion, halved and cut into
⅓-inch slices
2 tablespoons brown sugar

2 tablespoons balsamic vinegar
¼ cup chopped walnuts
6 cups fresh spinach

1. Heat the oil in a large skillet over medium heat.

2. Add the onion and sauté for 6 minutes, until it is translucent and softened.

3. Stir in the brown sugar and balsamic vinegar and continue to sauté 4 more minutes.

4. Stir in the walnuts and spinach, cover, and cook 2 minutes, until spinach is wilted.

5. Serve.

CHEF'S NOTE: If you're serving this salad as a main meal, don't forget to add your protein of choice. Salmon goes great with this recipe (see sheet pan recipe on page 61).

NUTRITION TIP: Walnuts may positively affect several health factors, including gut health, hunger and satiety, healthy aging, and metabolic health.

Per serving: Calories: 301; Total fat: 24g; Sodium: 82mg; Carbohydrates: 24g; Fiber: 4g; Sugar: 12g; Protein: 6g

ARTICHOKE WHITE BEAN ARUGULA SALAD

PREP TIME: 15 MINUTES | SERVES 2 (SERVING SIZE: 2 TABLESPOONS
DRESSING PLUS ALL OF THE SALAD INGREDIENTS)
30 MINUTES OR LESS | VEGETARIAN

If salad is going to be your main meal, it must contain all three macronutrients: carbohydrates, proteins, and fats. If salad is going to be a side or starter, eat the greens with another recipe from the lunch or dinner chapters. Salad does not have to be only greens; it can feature other vegetables like broccoli, spinach, or carrots. In this case, the headliner is artichokes.

For the lemon mustard vinaigrette

¼ cup freshly squeezed lemon juice

1 tablespoon extra-virgin olive oil

1 teaspoon Dijon mustard

½ teaspoon dried basil

½ teaspoon sea salt

¼ teaspoon freshly ground black pepper

For the salad

1 (14-ounce) can artichoke hearts, drained

1 (15-ounce) can white beans, drained and rinsed

4 cups arugula

2 ounces feta, crumbled

To make the lemon mustard vinaigrette

In a small bowl whisk the lemon juice, oil, mustard, basil, salt, and pepper until well combined.

To make the salad

1. Chop the artichoke hearts into bite-sized pieces, then toss them with the beans in a medium bowl.

2. Arrange the arugula on plates, top with the bean mixture, and sprinkle with the feta.

3. Just before serving, dress the salad with lemon mustard vinaigrette.

CHEF'S NOTE: Don't dress or season salads until you serve them because they can become soggy depending on the type of salad. Also, the leftovers keep in the refrigerator for up to 2 days.

NUTRITION TIP: Artichokes are good sources of fiber, vitamin C, folate, and magnesium.

Per serving: Calories: 310; Total fat: 7g; Sodium: 1,324mg; Carbohydrates: 43g; Fiber: 15g; Sugar: 6g; Protein: 18g

CORN SAUERKRAUT SALAD

PREP TIME: 15 MINUTES | SERVES 4 (SERVING SIZE: 1½ CUPS)
30 MINUTES OR LESS | VEGAN

A key ingredient in any salad is the fat. Fat can come in the form of oil, nuts, seeds, and avocado. Not only are these fats anti-inflammatory, but you need fat to absorb the fat-soluble vitamins (A, D, E, and K), antioxidants, and phytonutrients in vegetables. Add your protein of choice to this salad for a well-rounded meal.

3 (7-inch) carrots, thinly sliced
5 radishes, thinly sliced
1 (16-ounce) bag frozen corn, defrosted
1 (8-ounce) bag frozen peas, defrosted
¼ cup diced red onion

1 cup sauerkraut
2 tablespoons extra-virgin olive oil
3 tablespoons white wine vinegar
1½ teaspoons sea salt
½ teaspoon freshly ground black pepper

1. Place the carrots, radishes, corn, peas, onion, and sauerkraut in a medium bowl.

2. In a small bowl, whisk together the oil, vinegar, salt, and pepper until well blended.

3. Pour the dressing into the vegetable mixture and toss to combine.

4. Serve.

CHEF'S NOTE: To defrost frozen vegetables quicker, place them in a colander in the sink and rinse them with water for a couple minutes.

NUTRITION TIP: Sauerkraut is a fermented probiotic that eases digestion and improves gut health.

Per serving: Calories: 203; Total fat: 8g; Sodium: 1,191mg; Carbohydrates: 32g; Fiber: 7g; Sugar: 9g; Protein: 6g

AVOCADO MANGO SALAD

PREP TIME: 10 MINUTES | SERVES 2 (SERVING SIZE: 2 CUPS)
30 MINUTES OR LESS | ONE POT | VEGAN

Pairing mango with avocado is always a winner. Mangos are colorful and full of antioxidants. A 1-cup serving of mangos provides 30 percent of your daily vitamin A and 100 percent of your daily vitamin C.

1 mango, cubed
1 avocado, pitted, peeled, and cubed
1 cup cherry tomatoes, halved
½ cup diced red onion

2 tablespoons pine nuts
1 tablespoon freshly squeezed lemon juice
½ teaspoon sea salt

1. In a large bowl, toss together the mango, avocado, cherry tomatoes, onion, pine nuts, lemon juice, and sea salt until well mixed.

2. Serve.

CHEF'S NOTE: Grilled chicken or fish goes perfectly with this simple, colorful salad.

NUTRITION TIP: One-third of a medium avocado (50 g) has 80 calories and provides nearly 20 vitamins and minerals, making it a nutrient-rich choice.

Per serving: Calories: 302; Total fat: 20g; Sodium: 600mg; Carbohydrates: 34g; Fiber: 10g; Sugar: 19g; Protein: 5g

ROASTED BUTTERNUT AND QUINOA SALAD

PREP TIME: 10 MINUTES | COOK TIME: 25 MINUTES | SERVES 4 (SERVING SIZE: 1½ CUPS)
5 INGREDIENTS | ONE POT | VEGAN

Some salads are meant to be served immediately because the ingredients, like delicate watercress, are perishable when combined with dressing. However, other salads contain hearty grains and vegetables or taste better after several days of mellowing in the refrigerator. This filling salad is one that can be made ahead and eaten throughout the week.

4 cups butternut squash cubes
Nonstick cooking spray
Sea salt
2 cups Basic Quinoa (page 80)

1 cup frozen peas, defrosted
2 tablespoons minced fresh parsley
8 cups arugula

1. Preheat oven to 375°F.

2. Line a baking sheet with aluminum foil and arrange the squash cubes in a single layer on the sheet.

3. Coat the squash with cooking spray and season with salt. Roast the squash for 25 minutes or until tender.

4. Transfer the roasted squash to a medium bowl and add the quinoa, peas, and parsley. Toss to combine.

5. Evenly divide the arugula between four plates, top with the squash mixture, and serve.

> **CHEF'S NOTE:** This salad goes great with Parsley Tahini Dressing (see page 97) if you want to add some extra flavor to the dish.
>
> **NUTRITION TIP:** You can buy peeled and cut-up butternut squash at almost any supermarket. This can be a tremendous time-saver.

Per serving: Calories: 240; Total fat: 3g; Sodium: 63mg; Carbohydrates: 50g; Fiber: 12g; Sugar: 9g; Protein: 9g

ZESTY SHRIMP-STUFFED AVOCADO

PREP TIME: 10 MINUTES | SERVES 4 (SERVING SIZE: ½ STUFFED AVOCADO)
30 MINUTES OR LESS | ONE POT

Avocados are not only a superfood but a super serving vessel. I love to fill avocados with anything from eggs to tuna salads to quinoa. In this case, we are using chopped shrimp, sweet cherry tomatoes, and lots of fresh herbs. I recommend that you eat these avocados immediately, but if you can't, make sure you brush the outside and cut edges with lemon juice to delay browning.

8 ounces cooked, peeled, and deveined shrimp, chopped

2 scallions, thinly sliced (green and white parts)

1 cup cherry tomatoes, halved

⅓ cup chopped fresh cilantro

½ teaspoon sea salt

2 avocados, peeled, pitted, and halved

1. In a medium bowl, stir together the shrimp, scallions, tomatoes, cilantro, and salt until well mixed.

2. Evenly divide the filling among the avocado halves.

3. Serve immediately.

> **NUTRITION TIP:** Over 75 percent of the fat in avocados is unsaturated (monounsaturated and polyunsaturated fats), making them a great substitute for foods high in saturated fat.

Per serving: Calories: 212; Total fat: 14g; Sodium: 429mg; Carbohydrates: 10g; Fiber: 7g; Sugar: 2g; Protein: 14g

SUMPTUOUS SALMON SALAD

PREP TIME: 10 MINUTES | SERVES 4 (SERVING SIZE: 3 CUPS)
30 MINUTES OR LESS

This creation is a healthy twist on classic mayonnaise-drenched tuna salad. You can also scoop the salmon salad into sturdy Boston lettuce cups and use the chickpeas as a garnish for a simple and elegant presentation.

2 (6-ounce) cans wild-caught salmon, drained

2 (7-inch) celery stalks, thinly sliced

½ medium red onion, minced

½ cup chopped fresh parsley

¼ cup plus 2 tablespoons freshly squeezed lime juice

2 tablespoons extra-virgin olive oil

Sea salt

Freshly ground black pepper

6 cups fresh spinach

1 (15-ounce) can chickpeas, drained and rinsed

1. In a small bowl, mix together the salmon, celery, onion, parsley, lime juice, and oil until well combined. Season to taste with salt and pepper and set aside.

2. Place the spinach and beans in a large bowl and toss to combine.

3. Place the bean mixture on a serving plate, top with salmon salad, and serve.

NUTRITION TIP: This salad packs more nutritional power due to the abundant omega-3s found in salmon and monounsaturated fats from the extra-virgin olive oil.

Per serving: Calories: 316; Total fat: 16g; Sodium: 383mg; Carbohydrates: 25g; Fiber: 7g; Sugar: 5g; Protein: 21g

PARSLEY TAHINI DRESSING

PREP TIME: 5 MINUTES | SERVES 8 (SERVING SIZE: 2 TABLESPOONS)
30 MINUTES OR LESS | ONE POT | VEGAN

Based on many studies, the Mediterranean diet is by far one of the healthiest in the world. This lifestyle eating plan is bursting with lots of fruits, vegetables, nuts, and seeds like sesame seeds.

½ cup tahini, well stirred
6 tablespoons freshly squeezed lemon juice
2 tablespoons minced fresh parsley

1 tablespoon extra-virgin olive oil
½ teaspoon sea salt
¼ teaspoon freshly ground black pepper

1. In a medium bowl, whisk together the tahini, lemon juice, parsley, oil, salt, and pepper until smooth and well blended.

2. Store in the refrigerator until needed.

CHEF'S NOTE: This dressing can last 2 weeks refrigerated.

NUTRITION TIP: Tahini is a Mediterranean sesame paste similar in texture to peanut butter.

Per serving: Calories: 107; Total fat: 10g; Sodium: 166mg; Carbohydrates: 4g; Fiber: 2g; Sugar: <1g; Protein: 3g

MUSTARD LIME VINAIGRETTE

PREP TIME: 5 MINUTES | SERVES 4 (SERVING SIZE: ¼ CUP)
30 MINUTES OR LESS | ONE POT | VEGETARIAN

If you are looking for an all-purpose vinaigrette great for anything and everything, search no further. This simple dressing goes with every salad recipe in this book, and probably any salad your imagination can conjure up. Unfortunately, many dressings out there are loaded in fat. I made this one light and tasty.

½ cup freshly squeezed lime juice
2 tablespoons extra-virgin olive oil
1 teaspoon Dijon mustard

¼ teaspoon freshly ground black pepper
½ teaspoon dried basil
½ teaspoon sea salt

1. In a small bowl, whisk together the lime juice, oil, mustard, pepper, basil, and salt until well blended.

2. Let the dressing sit for 10 minutes.

3. Enjoy right away on a fresh salad or refrigerate for later, making sure to stir well before each use.

> **NUTRITION TIP:** This vinaigrette contains less fat than your common store-bought dressings therefore the serving size is ¼ cup rather than 2 tablespoons.

Per serving: Calories: 70; Total fat: 7g; Sodium: 321mg; Carbohydrates: 3g; Fiber: <1g; Sugar: 1g; Protein: <1g

LEMON BASIL YOGURT DRESSING

PREP TIME: 15 MINUTES | SERVES 4 (SERVING SIZE: ¼ CUP)
30 MINUTES OR LESS | ONE POT | VEGETARIAN

This dressing is one of those great recipes that can be easily changed to suit your palate. For example, if you prefer cilantro to basil and have a tasty Southwestern themed salad, simply use chopped cilantro in the same amount as the basil.

½ cup 2% plain Greek yogurt
¼ cup extra-virgin olive oil
2 tablespoons freshly squeezed lemon juice
2 tablespoons chopped fresh basil or cilantro

½ teaspoon minced garlic
¼ teaspoon sea salt
¼ teaspoon black pepper

1. In a small bowl, whisk together the yogurt, oil, lemon juice, basil, garlic, salt, and pepper until well blended.

2. Let sit for 10 minutes. Enjoy right away or refrigerate for later, making sure to stir well before each use.

NUTRITION TIP: Most people seek flavor through dressing, so having one made with herbs is even more flavorful than oil-based ones.

Per serving: Calories: 144; Total fat: 14g; Sodium: 156mg; Carbohydrates: 2g; Fiber: <1g; Sugar: 1g; Protein: 3g

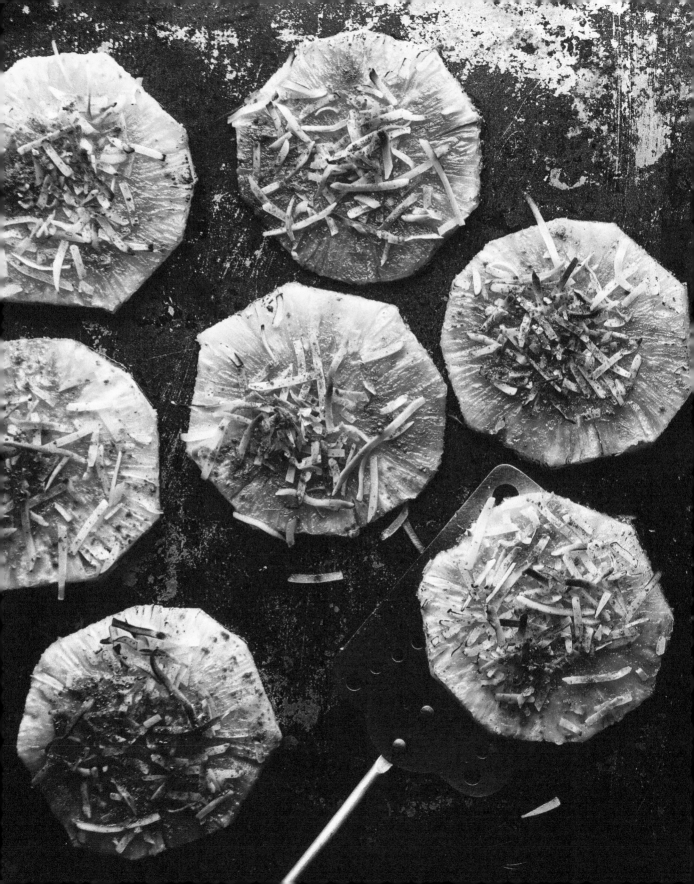

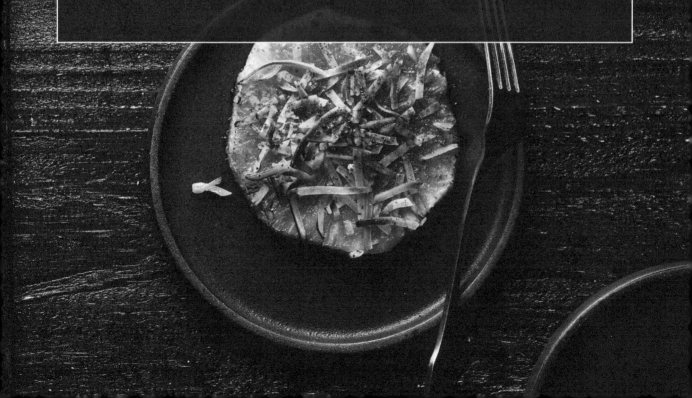

CHAPTER EIGHT

DESSERTS

This is probably my favorite chapter because, even as a registered dietitian, I absolutely love sweets. In this culture desserts are often looked at as evil, but on the contrary, they can be a key part of a healthy lifestyle so long as you use the right ingredients, as the recipes in this chapter do. Many of these desserts use fruit and dark chocolate, which are superfoods that offer nutrients and antioxidants to fight inflammation, along with adding some indulgence. What a sweet deal!

ROASTED COCONUT PINEAPPLE

PREP TIME: 5 MINUTES | COOK TIME: 25 MINUTES | SERVES 8 (SERVING SIZE: 1 SLICE)
5 INGREDIENTS | ONE POT | VEGAN

Using fresh fruit to make dessert is a win-win in taste and nutrition. Not only do you get a serving of fruit, you also get a satisfying hit of sweetness.

Nonstick cooking spray

1 pineapple, peeled, sliced into 8 (½-inch) rounds, and cored

8 tablespoons dried flaked unsweetened coconut

Sea salt

Ground cinnamon

8 teaspoons coconut sugar

1. Preheat oven to 450°F.

2. Line a baking sheet with aluminum foil and coat with cooking spray.

3. Place the pineapple slices in a single layer on the prepared baking sheet. Sprinkle each slice with a tablespoon of coconut, a pinch of salt, a pinch of cinnamon, and 1 teaspoon of coconut sugar.

4. Bake for 25 minutes.

5. Serve.

CHEF'S NOTE: Sometimes, even sweet things need a little bit of salt. Here, a sprinkle of sea salt really brings out the flavor of the pineapple.

NUTRITION TIP: Roasting the pineapple is a great way to caramelize the natural sugars and deepen the flavors. Peaches and nectarines are also good choices for roasting.

Per serving: Calories: 79; Total fat: 4g; Sodium: 2mg; Carbohydrates: 12g; Fiber: 1g; Sugar: 10g; Protein: 1g

NO BAKE CREAMY LIME CHEESECAKE

PREP TIME: 20 MINUTES, PLUS 30 MINUTES TO CHILL | SERVES 4 (SERVING SIZE: 1 SQUARE 2-INCH SLICE)
30 MINUTES OR LESS | VEGETARIAN

By far, key lime pie is my favorite American dessert. Unfortunately, the traditional recipe for this tart, creamy dish calls for sugar-packed condensed milk. I needed to make a lighter version that I can enjoy regularly, and I succeeded. I'm here to share my key lime love affair with you.

8 ounces light cream cheese
½ cup 2% plain Greek yogurt
5 tablespoons freshly squeezed lime juice

¼ cup sugar
6 graham crackers
1 teaspoon lime zest

1. Soften the cream cheese in the microwave for 30 seconds.

2. Transfer the cream cheese to a medium bowl and whisk in the yogurt, lime juice, and sugar until well blended.

3. Crumble the graham crackers into the bottom of an 8-by-8-inch baking dish.

4. Spread the cream cheese mixture over the crumbs.

5. Sprinkle the lime zest on the cream cheese.

6. Refrigerate for 30 minutes to set and cut into squares.

7. Serve.

CHEF'S NOTE: Refrigerate the leftovers for up to 3 days.

NUTRITION TIP: Substituting full-fat cream cheese for light cream cheese helps to reduce the calories of this dessert. Same goes with just adding sugar instead of using a whole can of condensed milk.

Per serving: Calories: 305; Total fat: 15g; Sodium: 350mg; Carbohydrates: 30g; Fiber: 1g; Sugar: 19g; Protein: 8g

STRAWBERRIES AND CREAM CHIA PUDDING

PREP TIME: 10 MINUTES, PLUS 3 HOURS TO CHILL | SERVES 4 (SERVING SIZE: ¼ CUP)
5 INGREDIENTS | 30 MINUTES OR LESS | VEGETARIAN

Here is a delicious dessert that allows you to enjoy the yummy flavors and creamy texture of pudding without any cream at all. Chia seeds provide the thick pudding-like consistency and a hefty amount of nutrients like omega-3s, calcium, and protein. For a real treat, top this pale pink dessert with a scoop of whipped coconut cream.

2 cups whole cow's milk

2 cups strawberries, hulled

6 tablespoons chia seeds

2 tablespoons honey

1. Place the milk and strawberries in a blender and blend until smooth.

2. Pour the blended liquid into a container with a lid.

3. Stir in the chia seeds and honey until well mixed.

4. Put the lid on the container and refrigerate for 3 hours until it thickens into a pudding consistency.

5. Serve.

> **NUTRITION TIP:** One serving of 8 medium California strawberries provides 110 percent of your recommended daily value of vitamin C, which is a potent antioxidant. The same amount also provides 5 percent of your daily value of potassium, a nutrient that helps balance electrolytes, aid muscle contractions, and maintain a healthy blood pressure. Also, 8 medium strawberries a day provides 3 grams of fiber, making this fruit a good source of dietary fiber.

Per serving: Calories: 219; Total fat: 9g; Sodium: 61mg; Carbohydrates: 27g; Fiber: 9g; Sugar: 18g; Protein: 9g

BAKED APPLES WITH CINNAMON

PREP TIME: 20 MINUTES | COOK TIME: 30 MINUTES | SERVES 4 (SERVING SIZE: 1 APPLE HALF)
5 INGREDIENTS | ONE POT | VEGAN

Looking for another way to improve your fruit intake while enjoying a delicious dessert? Try tender cinnamon-scented baked apples with a satisfying nutty crunch.

2 sweet apples (Pink Lady or
Fuji work nicely), halved

4 teaspoons chopped walnuts

4 teaspoons brown sugar

Ground cinnamon, for sprinkling

1. Preheat oven to 400°F.

2. Line a baking dish with aluminum foil and set aside.

3. Core each apple half with a paring knife.

4. Top each apple half with 1 teaspoon of walnuts and 1 teaspoon of brown sugar. Sprinkle each with ground cinnamon.

5. Place the apples in the prepared baking dish and cover the dish with foil.

6. Bake the apples for 30 minutes or until tender.

7. Serve warm.

> **CHEF'S TIP:** The best time to make this simple dessert is in the fall when apples are in season and there is a great selection of varieties to try.

Per serving: Calories: 75; Total fat: 2g; Sodium: 2mg; Carbohydrates: 17g; Fiber: 2g; Sugar: 12g; Protein: 1g

SEA SALT CARAMEL FUDGE BROWNIES

PREP TIME: 10 MINUTES | COOK TIME: 15 MINUTES | SERVES 16 (SERVING SIZE: 2-INCH SQUARE)
30 MINUTES OR LESS | VEGETARIAN

You might notice this recipe uses cacao powder instead of cocoa powder; they are different products. Cacao powder is made from cold-pressed raw cacao beans, and cocoa powder is made from beans that have been toasted at high temperatures. Cacao powder contains live enzymes and more nutrients.

Nonstick cooking spray
1 cup all-purpose flour
½ cup cacao powder
¼ cup brown sugar
¼ teaspoon sea salt
⅔ cup whole cow's milk

1 large egg
2 large egg yolks
1 teaspoon vanilla extract
1 (3½-ounce) dark chocolate bar
    filled with caramel, chopped
¼ cup unsweetened shredded coconut
¼ cup chopped walnuts

1. Preheat oven to 350°F.

2. Lightly coat an 8-by-8-inch baking dish with cooking spray.

3. In a medium bowl, stir together the flour, cacao powder, brown sugar, and salt until well combined.

4. In a small bowl, whisk together the milk, egg, egg yolks, and vanilla until blended.

5. Add the egg mixture to the flour mixture and stir until just combined.

6. Stir in the chocolate, coconut, and walnuts until just mixed.

7. Spoon the batter into the prepared baking dish and bake 15 minutes or until a toothpick inserted in the center comes out clean.

8. Cool and serve.

> **CHEF'S TIP:** Beware, these fudge brownies are way too delicious so you might end up eating them all yourself instead of sharing. Eat them mindfully!

Per serving: Calories: 96; Total fat: 4g; Sodium: 51mg; Carbohydrates: 13g; Fiber: 2g; Sugar: 4g; Protein: 3g

DARK CHOCOLATE MIXED DRIED FRUIT

PREP TIME: 20 MINUTES, PLUS 20 MINUTES TO FREEZE | COOK TIME: 1½ MINUTES | SERVES 4
(SERVING SIZE: 3 PIECES)
30 MINUTES OR LESS | VEGAN

Sometimes a couple of simple ingredients create a delicious finished product that is near perfect. Slightly bitter dark chocolate highlights the natural concentrated sweetness of dried fruit and the hint of salt creates magic. Make this recipe over the weekend and store the dried fruit as a pick-me-up treat or dessert during the week.

3½ ounces 73% dark chocolate,
  finely chopped
Pinch sea salt
3 dried figs

3 dates
3 dried apricots
3 prunes

1. Line a small baking sheet with parchment paper and set aside.

2. Place the chocolate in a small bowl and microwave 1½ minutes in three separate 30-second intervals, stirring in between each. Stir in the salt.

3. Dip the dried figs, dates, apricots, and prunes in the melted chocolate. Place the dipped fruit on the prepared baking sheet and freeze for about 20 minutes to harden.

4. Serve.

CHEF'S NOTE: To store, refrigerate the dipped fruit to keep the chocolate from melting.

NUTRITION TIP: Eating dried fruit counts toward your daily intake of fruits for the day.

Per serving: Calories: 216; Total fat: 9g; Sodium: 2mg; Carbohydrates: 32g; Fiber: 6g; Sugar: 23g; Protein: 1g

MANGO SOUR FROZEN YOGURT

PREP TIME: 10 MINUTES, PLUS 3 HOURS TO FREEZE | SERVES 4 (SERVING SIZE: ¼ CUP)
5 INGREDIENTS | 30 MINUTES OR LESS | VEGETARIAN

If you are a frozen yogurt aficionado, you will love this homemade version and be amazed that it is so easy to make without any complicated techniques or equipment. You can use an ice cream maker if you already own one and just follow the manufacturer's instructions, but the blend, freeze, and scoop method works fine.

2 cups fresh mango chunks
(2 medium mangos)

1 cup 2% plain Greek yogurt
2 tablespoons honey

1. Place the mango, yogurt, and honey in a food processor or blender and purée until creamy.

2. Transfer the mixture to a container with a lid.

3. Place the container in the freezer for about 3 hours and serve.

CHEF'S NOTE: You can freeze this dessert for up to 1 week. If the mixture freezes too hard to scoop, let it sit at room temperature for about 10 minutes to thaw slightly before serving.

NUTRITION TIP: You can also use this frozen yogurt as your preworkout shake, just add protein powder and some more milk and blend.

Per serving: Calories: 128; Total fat: 2g; Sodium: 28mg; Carbohydrates: 25g; Fiber: 2g; Sugar: 22g; Protein: 6g

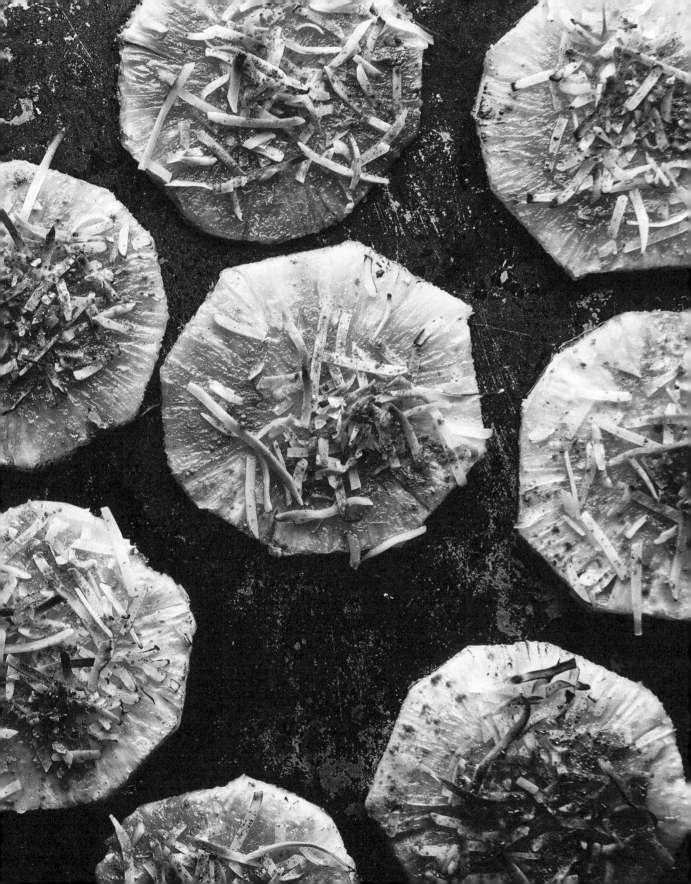

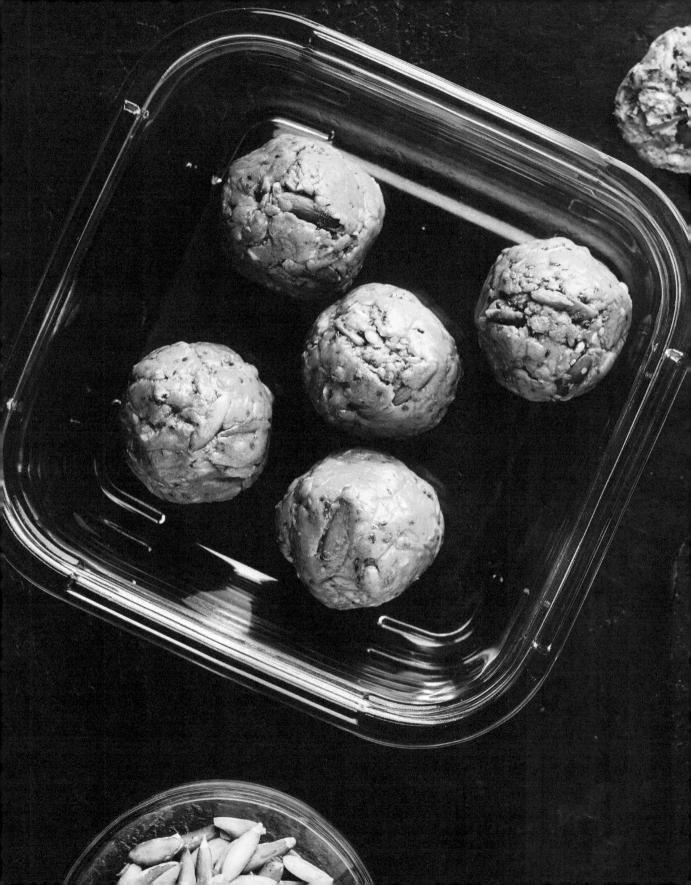

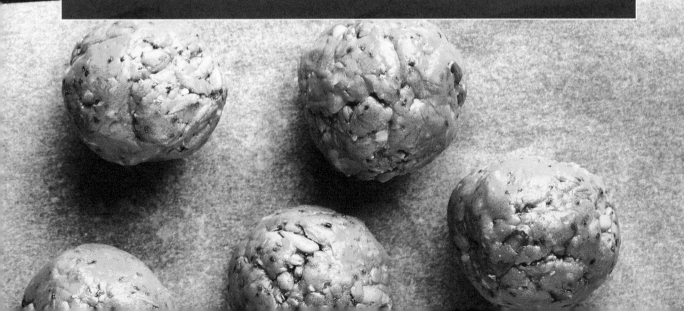

CHAPTER NINE

HEARTY SNACKS

Snacks are a crucial part of keeping your hunger in check. Think about it: Your lunch break at work was around noon and you don't get home until six. By then you're starving and end up having two dinners along with the cheese, crackers, and chips in between. That's why including snacks that contain a good amount of protein for satiety between meals is vital to keep you from eating more than you should later. I always recommend a midafternoon snack (between 3:00 and 5:00 p.m.) like the ones in this chapter to keep you from overeating at dinner and your other main meals.

APPLE AND EGGS

PREP TIME: 5 MINUTES | SERVES 1
5 INGREDIENTS | 30 MINUTES OR LESS | ONE POT | VEGETARIAN

You might be asking yourself what is so special about apple and egg. There is culinary synchronicity in these two ingredients because they taste great and will help you follow a healthy lifestyle. One way to curb your appetite and not overeat at dinner is to have an afternoon snack around 3:00 or 4:00 p.m. Including a carbohydrate (apple in this case) and protein (hard-boiled egg) ensures satiation.

2 hard-boiled eggs, sliced

1 apple, sliced

Eat the eggs and apple at the same time for a satisfying snack.

CHEF'S TIP: Put the apple slices in a sealable plastic bag with 1 teaspoon freshly squeezed lime juice to keep the fruit from browning.

Per serving: Calories: 251; Total fat: 11g; Sodium: 126mg; Carbohydrates: 26g; Fiber: 4g; Sugar: 20g; Protein: 13g

POWER PACKED TRAIL MIX

PREP TIME: 5 MINUTES | SERVES 4 (SERVING SIZE: ½ CUP)
5 INGREDIENTS | 30 MINUTES OR LESS | ONE POT | VEGAN

Store-bought trail mixes have added sugars and other ingredients you probably cannot pronounce and certainly don't want to eat. Thankfully, it's so much easier and cheaper to make your own.

½ cup cocoa nibs
½ cup dried unsweetened blueberries

½ cup unsweetened dried flaked coconut
½ cup roasted salted almonds

1. Stir together the cocoa nibs, blueberries, coconut, and almonds in a medium bowl until well mixed.

2. Transfer to a container with a lid and store in pantry.

CHEF'S NOTE: Eat it within 1 week.

NUTRITION TIP: The specific ingredients are not important. If you like dried cranberries, cashews, walnuts, or sunflower seeds instead, feel free to experiment.

Per serving: Calories: 573; Total fat: 29g; Sodium: 124mg; Carbohydrates: 73g; Fiber: 13g; Sugar: 5g; Protein: 6g

AVOCADO TOAST WITH TURKEY

PREP TIME: 5 MINUTES | SERVES 1
5 INGREDIENTS | 30 MINUTES OR LESS | ONE POT

Avocado toast is one of those dishes that seems to be everywhere these days; everyone is making it! Many people reserve this combination for breakfast because that is where you usually find toast, but it can be enjoyed as a filling snack as well. The added turkey provides a nice hit of protein to the healthy fats and carbs.

1 slice whole-grain bread

½ very ripe avocado

2 ounces sliced deli turkey

1. Toast the bread.

2. Mash the avocado onto the bread using a fork, top with the turkey, and enjoy.

NUTRITION TIP: Avocados contain 136 micrograms of lutein and zeaxanthin per 50-gram serving (one-third of a medium avocado). Lutein and zeaxanthin are carotenoids that some research suggests may help maintain eye health as we age.

Per serving: Calories: 314; Total fat: 16g; Sodium: 637mg; Carbohydrates: 31g; Fiber: 11g; Sugar: 5g; Protein: 19g

GREEK YOGURT WITH STRAWBERRIES

PREP TIME: 5 MINUTES | SERVES 1
5 INGREDIENTS | 30 MINUTES OR LESS | ONE POT | VEGETARIAN

I call this snack a triple-winner. You get antioxidants from fruit, probiotics from yogurt, and monounsaturated fats from walnuts. This combination will definitely leave you satisfied and tastes amazing.

1 cup 2% plain Greek yogurt

½ cup sliced strawberries

2 tablespoons chopped walnuts

Layer the yogurt, strawberries, and walnuts in a bowl and enjoy.

> **CHEF'S TIP:** California strawberries are best when consumed in season when they are sweet and their fragrance can fill the kitchen. The peak season for these bright berries is April through June, but they are available year-round.

Per serving: Calories: 345; Total fat: 24g; Sodium: 151mg; Carbohydrates: 35g; Fiber: 12g; Sugar: 5g; Protein: 12g

TURKEY SPINACH ROLL

PREP TIME: 15 MINUTES | SERVES 1
5 INGREDIENTS | 30 MINUTES OR LESS | ONE POT

When clients ask me, "What is the perfect snack, Manuel?" I say, "Sometimes it can be a mini-meal." What is a mini-meal? It's carbs, fats, protein, and greens all in one handy package. This wrap is your perfect mini-meal snack when you need a boost during the day.

1 (10-by-8-inch) piece lavash bread

1 tablespoon avocado oil mayonnaise

4 ounces deli turkey

½ cup packed fresh spinach

1. Spread the mayonnaise on the lavash bread to about 1 inch from the edges.

2. Place the turkey over a third of the bread and top with the spinach. Roll the bread into a wrap starting at the short end, cut in half, and enjoy.

> **NUTRITION TIP:** Always try to include vegetables when you can.

Per serving: Calories: 304; Total fat: 35g; Sodium: 1,557mg; Carbohydrates: 15g; Fiber: 6g; Sugar: <1g; Protein: 28g

YOGURT BERRY PROTEIN SMOOTHIE

PREP TIME: 5 MINUTES | SERVES 1
5 INGREDIENTS | 30 MINUTES OR LESS | ONE POT | VEGETARIAN

Working from home today? Make this smoothie as your snack to provide the perfect pick-me-up for that inevitable morning energy slump! Or prepare it in advance and have it in the midafternoon between tasks. You will enjoy it whenever you choose to consume this tangy, sweet snack.

1 cup 2% plain Greek yogurt
1 cup berries (strawberries, blueberries, raspberries)

1 cup whole milk (or milk of choice)
1 scoop protein powder* (whey, soy, pea, or rice)
Note: To provide 25 grams of protein

Place the yogurt, berries, milk, and protein powder in a blender and blend until smooth and enjoy.

NUTRITION TIP: Cow's milk helps with both pre- and post-exercise fueling. Not only does it have protein and carbohydrates, but it also contains branched chain amino acids (valine, isoleucine, and leucine), which are essential for post-exercise recovery.

Per serving: Calories: 526; Total fat: 23g; Sodium: 422mg; Carbohydrates: 39g; Fiber: 4g; Sugar: 33g; Protein: 43g

GUT-HEALTHY HUMMUS WITH VEGETABLES

PREP TIME: 10 MINUTES | SERVES 3 (SERVING SIZE: ¼ CUP)
30 MINUTES OR LESS | ONE POT | VEGETARIAN

Kefir is a fermented milk drink high in protein, so it really fills you up. This product is not a traditional ingredient in hummus, but it adds a tanginess and amazing creamy texture. Once you taste this recipe, you might decide to add it to other dips and sauces.

1 (15-ounce) can chickpeas, rinsed and drained

½ cup plain unsweetened kefir

1 tablespoon freshly squeezed lemon juice

½ teaspoon sea salt

¼ teaspoon garlic powder

¼ teaspoon freshly ground black pepper

Carrots, bell peppers, celery, or other crudités of choice, for serving

1. Place the chickpeas, kefir, lemon juice, salt, garlic powder, and pepper in a food processor and purée until the desired texture.

2. Serve with the vegetables.

NUTRITION TIP: In this recipe, kefir takes the place of tahini, which is the traditional ingredient used in hummus. You might lose a little of the rich flavor, but kefir brings gut-friendly probiotics into the mix.

Per serving: Calories: 184; Total fat: 3g; Sodium: 415mg; Carbohydrates: 30g; Fiber: 7g; Sugar: 7g; Protein: 10g

ROASTED VEGETABLE SOUP TO GO

PREP TIME: 5 MINUTES | SERVES 4 (SERVING SIZE: 2 CUPS)
5 INGREDIENTS | 30 MINUTES OR LESS | ONE POT | VEGAN

Snacks don't have to be complicated or even solid! Soup is a perfect grab and go choice that can fill you up and provide valuable nutrients and energy to get you through a busy day.

2 cups Basic Roasted Vegetables (page 81)

1 cup low-sodium vegetable or chicken stock

1. Place the vegetables and stock in a blender and blend until the desired texture.

2. Pour the soup into a to-go container and enjoy during the day.

> **NUTRITION TIP:** Pair this soup with a chunk of cheese or hard-boiled egg to provide a protein source.

Per serving: Calories: 39; Total fat: 2g; Sodium: 270mg; Carbohydrates: 5g; Fiber: 2g; Sugar: 2g; Protein: 1g

KICK-ASS PREWORKOUT PROTEIN MUFFINS

PREP TIME: 15 MINUTES | **COOK TIME: 20 MINUTES** | **SERVES 12 (SERVING SIZE: 1 MUFFIN)**
VEGETARIAN

As a registered dietitian, one mistake I see a lot of male clients make is they exercise without fueling correctly. This muffin makes a great preworkout snack. It provides good carbohydrates and protein essential for success in the gym or on the field or court. You can freeze these muffins individually in sealable plastic bags for a convenient snack all week.

Nonstick cooking spray
2 cups all-purpose flour
2 scoops vanilla protein powder*
  (whey, soy, pea, or rice)
1 teaspoon baking soda
1 teaspoon baking powder
1 teaspoon sea salt
3 medium ripe bananas, mashed

2 large eggs
½ cup 2% plain Greek yogurt
¼ cup canola oil
¼ cup whole cow's milk
1 teaspoon vanilla extract
10 prunes, finely chopped
Note: To provide 25 grams of protein

1. Preheat oven to 350°F.

2. Line a 12-cup muffin tin with paper cups and coat with cooking spray.

3. In a large bowl, whisk the flour, protein powder, baking soda, baking powder, and salt until well blended. Set aside.

4. In a medium bowl, whisk together the mashed bananas, eggs, yogurt, oil, milk, and vanilla until well mixed.

5. Pour the wet ingredients into the dry ingredients and stir until just combined. Stir in the prunes.

6. Spoon the batter into the prepared muffin cups and bake for 20 minutes, or until a toothpick inserted in the center comes out clean.

7. Serve.

CHEF'S NOTE: Be careful not to over-stir the batter because this will develop the gluten, making the muffins tough. Stir just until the flour is absorbed.

NUTRITION TIP: Pair the muffin with a glass of milk as your pre-exercise fuel.

Per serving: Calories: 192; Total fat: 6g; Sodium: 342mg; Carbohydrates: 27g; Fiber: 2g; Sugar: 7g; Protein: 9g

NO BAKE SEED BITES

PREP TIME: 5 MINUTES | SERVES 6 (SERVING SIZE: 2 BALLS)
30 MINUTES OR LESS | VEGETARIAN

WARNING: Too delicious! Keep these sweet and rich treats on hand as a favorite snack and try to enjoy only two at a time, if possible. The recipe calls for chocolate protein powder, but vanilla will also be delicious with the seeds and sweet honey.

1 cup peanut butter or almond butter
2 tablespoons roasted pumpkin seeds
2 tablespoons chia seeds
2 tablespoons flaxseed
2 tablespoons roasted sunflower seeds

1 tablespoon honey
½ cup quick one-minute oats
1 scoop chocolate protein powder
   (whey, soy, pea, or rice)
Note: To provide 25 grams of protein

1. In a large bowl, stir together the peanut butter, pumpkin seeds, chia seeds, flaxseed, sunflower seeds, and honey until well mixed.

2. Stir in the oats and protein powder until well combined.

3. When the mixture starts looking dry, knead with your hands to form one giant ball.

4. Scoop the mixture into 12 equally sized balls (about 1 ounce or 2 tablespoons per ball).

5. Transfer to a container with a lid and refrigerate until very firm.

> **NUTRITION TIP:** Seeds are nutritional powerhouses, packed with abundant minerals, vitamins, and nutrients.

Per serving: Calories: 368; Total fat: 26g; Sodium: 231mg; Carbohydrates: 20g; Fiber: 7g; Sugar: 8g; Protein: 18g

RECOMMENDED FOOD BRANDS

Throughout the book I have mentioned a variety of foods that I include in my everyday diet from fruit and condiments to bread and pasta, and my clients in my private practice frequently ask for brand recommendations. I've made it simple for you by including a list of my favorite brands and food commodities here. Keep in mind that I am a spokesperson for some of the brands included, but I only represent brands that I use personally, brands that I believe in and that align with my personal morals and philosophies as a registered dietitian.

- Atoria's Family Bakery (lavash, naan, flatbreads)

- Barilla ProteinPlus pasta

- California Almonds

- California Avocados

- California Figs

- California Strawberries

- California Walnuts

- Chobani yogurts

- Dave's Killer Bread

- Green Valley Creamery (lactose-free products)

- Hellmann's Avocado Oil Mayonnaise

- Quaker Oats

- Sunsweet Amaz!n Prunes

MEASUREMENT CONVERSIONS

	US STANDARD	US STANDARD (OUNCES)	METRIC (APPROXIMATE)
VOLUME EQUIVALENTS (LIQUID)	2 tablespoons	1 fl. oz.	30 mL
	¼ cup	2 fl. oz.	60 mL
	½ cup	4 fl. oz.	120 mL
	1 cup	8 fl. oz.	240 mL
	1½ cups	12 fl. oz.	355 mL
	2 cups or 1 pint	16 fl. oz.	475 mL
	4 cups or 1 quart	32 fl. oz.	1 L
	1 gallon	128 fl. oz.	4 L
VOLUME EQUIVALENTS (DRY)	⅛ teaspoon		0.5 mL
	¼ teaspoon		1 mL
	½ teaspoon		2 mL
	¾ teaspoon		4 mL
	1 teaspoon		5 mL
	1 tablespoon		15 mL
	¼ cup		59 mL
	⅓ cup		79 mL
	½ cup		118 mL
	⅔ cup		156 mL
	¾ cup		177 mL
	1 cup		235 mL
	2 cups or 1 pint		475 mL
	3 cups		700 mL
	4 cups or 1 quart		1 L
	½ gallon		2 L
	1 gallon		4 L
WEIGHT EQUIVALENTS	½ ounce		15 g
	1 ounce		30 g
	2 ounces		60 g
	4 ounces		115 g
	8 ounces		225 g
	12 ounces		340 g
	16 ounces or 1 pound		455 g

	FAHRENHEIT (F)	CELSIUS (C) (APPROXIMATE)
OVEN TEMPERATURES	250°F	120°F
	300°F	150°C
	325°F	180°C
	375°F	190°C
	400°F	200°C
	425°F	220°C
	450°F	230°C

INDEX

ACKNOWLEDGMENTS

I want to especially thank Destini Moody for her writing contributions, Alejandro Pinot and Maggie Taylor for recipe development assistance, and my husband, Jeff, for recipe tasting.

ABOUT THE AUTHOR

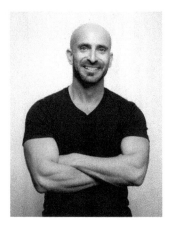

Manuel Villacorta, MS, RD, is an internationally recognized, award-winning registered dietitian-nutritionist with more than eighteen years of experience. He is the author of four nutrition, wellness, and weight loss books. Villacorta is a trusted voice in the health and wellness industry. His knowledge, charismatic talent, and bilingual proficiency in English and Spanish have made him an in-demand health and nutrition expert on local and national television, as well as on radio.

He acts as a national spokesperson/ambassador who represents food commodities and recognized brands such as California Avocados, California Strawberries, the National Mango Board, the American Egg Board, Unilever, the National Dairy Council, the US Canola Oil Association, Pichuberry, a2 Milk, Green Valley Creamery, Foster Farms, the National Pork Board, Sunsweet Amaz!n Prunes, and Quaker Oats, among others.

He is one of the leading weight loss and nutrition experts in the country. Manuel is the owner of MV Nutrition, a San Francisco–based private practice, and the recipient of five "Best Bay Area Nutritionist" awards from the *San Francisco Chronicle*, ABC7 News, and Citysearch. Manuel was featured and recognized for his contributions and as a preeminent Latino registered dietitian nutritionist in the San Francisco Bay area by ABC7, a leading media outlet in the region.

Born and raised in Peru, he currently lives in San Francisco. Villacorta earned his bachelor of science in nutrition and physiology metabolism from the University of California, Berkeley, and his master of science in nutrition and food science from California State University, San Jose. He has been the recipient of numerous prestigious awards for his research and contributions to the field of nutrition and dietetics, including: First Place Award Winner in the category of Health, Nutrition, and Clinical Science at the 18th annual statewide student research competition among the California State universities, Outstanding Researcher Award by Graduate Studies and Research at San Jose State University, and the Emerging Dietetic Leader Award by The Academy of Nutrition and Dietetics.

CPSIA information can be obtained
at www.ICGtesting.com
Printed in the USA
BVHW090717071120
592607BV00004B/8